AF526876

DM ENDOCRINOLOGY ENTRANCE EXAMINATION

(Includes Important Text, Original solved MCQ's and their Explanations)

DM ENDOCRINOLOGY ENTRANCE EXAMINATION

(Includes Important Text, Original solved MCQ's and their Explanations)

Editor :
Dr. M.S. Bhatia (M.D.; MNAMS)
Prof & Head, Department of Psychiatry
University College of Medical Sciences &
Guru Teg Bahadur Hospital,
Dilshad Garden Delhi - 110095,

Contributing Editor :
Dr. (Mrs.) Nirmaljit Kaur (M.D.)
Senior Specialist, Department of Microbiology
Dr. R.M.L., Hospital
New Delhi - 110001

CBS

CBS Publishers & Distributors Pvt. Ltd.

New Delhi • Bengaluru • Chennai • Kochi • Kolkata • Mumbai
Hyderabad • Nagpur • Patna • Pune • Vijayawada

Dedicated to

Respected Teachers & Beloved Students

ISBN: 81-239-1352-4

First Edition: 2006
Reprint: 2007, 2010, 2013, 2016, 2018

Published by **Satish Kumar Jain** and produced by **Varun Jain** for
CBS Publishers & Distributors Pvt. Ltd.,
4819/XI Prahlad Street, 24 Ansari Road, Daryaganj, New Delhi - 110002
delhi@cbspd.com, cbspubs@airtelmail.in • www.cbspd.com
Ph.: 23289259, 23266861, 23266867 • Fax: 011-23243014

Corporate Office: 204 FIE, Industrial Area, Patparganj, Delhi - 110 092
Ph: 49344934 • Fax: 011-49344935
E-mail: publishing@cbspd.com • publicity@cbspd.com

Branches:
- ***Bengaluru:*** 2975, 17th Cross, K.R. Road, Bansankari 2nd Stage, Bengaluru - 70 • Ph: +91-80-26771678/79 • Fax: +91-80-26771680 E-mail: cbsbng@gmail.com, bangalore@cbspd.com
- ***Chennai:*** No. 7, Subbaraya Street, Shenoy Nagar, Chennai - 600030 Ph: +91-44-26681266, 26680620 • Fax: +91-44-42032115 E-mail: chennai@cbspd.com
- ***Kochi:*** Ashana House, 39/1904, A.M. Thomas Road, Valanjambalam, Ernakulum, Kochi • Ph: +91-484-4059061-65 Fax: +91-484-4059065 • E-mail: cochin@cbspd.com
- ***Kolkata:*** 6-B, Ground Floor, Rameshwar Shaw Road, Kolkata - 700014 Ph: +91-33-22891126/7/8 • E-mail: kolkata@cbspd.com
- ***Mumbai:*** 83-C, Dr. E. Moses Road, Worli, Mumbai - 400018 Ph: +91-9833017933, 022-24902340/41 • E-mail: mumbai@cbspd.com

Representatives:
- Hyderabad: 0-9885175004
- Patna: 0-9334159340
- Jharkhand: 0-9811541605
- Nagpur: 0-9021734563
- Pune: 0-9623451994
- Uttarakhand: 0-9716462459

Printed at: J.S. Offset Printers, Delhi (India)

PREFACE

Medical science is a rapidly advancing field. Its new allied branches are coming up. In a competitive examination, more and more emphasis is being laid on these allied disciplines. But most of the standard textbooks of surgery have failed to devote adequate space to these new disciplines.

This book has been written with the aim to outline the major areas of Endocrinology i.e Factual data, Commonest symptoms or cause, Named signs and syndromes and *Recent advances.* This book is not merely an addition to the existing list of books on MCQ's but a sincere ambition and an honest attempt to make it a useful and practical companion to both medical graduates and postgraduates. The present book consists of original solved MCQ's from the *Question Banks* of various important examinations (AIIMS, Delhi, PGI etc.), Important text, original solved MCQ's and their explanations have been added. I hope that this will help the candidates in performing better in the examination.

All suggestions for the modification of this book are welcome and will be duly acknowledged.

—Editors

CONTENTS

IMPORTANT TEXT OF ENDOCRINOLOGY

IMPORTANT POINTS TO REMEMBER

* Pituitary gland : **13 x 8 mm.**
* **Thyroid gland measures :**
  Lobes **5 x 2.5 x 2.5 cm.**
  Isthmus **3.7 x 1.2 cm.**
* **C-cells** in thyroid gland are derived from Ultimobranchial body.
* Thyroid gland is attached to cartilages of larynx by —Pretracheal fascia.
* Pancreas is retroperitoneal organ.
* Pancreatic islets are more abundant in the tail of the pancreas and contain α cells which secrete glucogen; β cells which secrete insulin; γ cells secrete somatostatin which inhibits secretory activity of β or more a α cells.
* δ_1 and PP cells are not confined to islets but distributed to many exocrine tissues of pancreas.
* GEP (Gastro Entero Pancreatic) endocrine system belongs to APUD cell series and has scattered solitary hormone producing cells in gastrointestinal mucosa and pancreas.
* Superior thyroid artery is related to external laryngeal nerve. Nerve lies frequently on a more posterior plane.
* An adult pancreas has **2.5-7.5 lac** islets.
* Metyrapone inhibits **11-beta hydroxylase.**
* Testosterone increases BMR by **15%** by increasing protein anabolism.
* Testosterone causes an increase in **RBC** by **20%.**
* Severe stress can raise ACTH and cortisol level by **20 folds.**
* Hyperthyroidism increases BMR **60 to 100%** above normal while hypothyroidism may decrease it to **30 to 45%.**
* Steroid hormones and T3, T4 act by enhancing specific protein synthesis and thus require **30-45 minutes** for its action to start.
* Amino acid content of some polypeptide hormones

GH 191	
Somatomedin (C)	70
IGF-II	67
Somatostatin	14
Oxytocin/ADH	9

* Maximum GH secretion occurs **2 hours** after falling asleep.
* SIADH is characterized by low Na^+ in extracellular fluids(less than **130 meq per litre).**
* ACTH secretion is **maximum** between 1.00a.m. to 4.00a.m. and **minimum** at about one hour after falling asleep.
* The catecholamines, which are converted to VMA are 30%
* Of circulating T3, **80%** is derived from deiodinated T_4
* Weight of pituitary is about **0.5 gm**
* Half life of GH is **20-30 minutes**
* Normal concentration of GH in plasma in can adults is **3 multi m μg/ml (6 milli μg/ml** in a child)
* Vasopressin differs from oxytocin by 2 amino acids (i.e. Vasopression has arginine and phenylalanine out of 8 aminoacids whereas oxytocin has leucine and isoleucine)
* Removal of thyroid causes decrease in BMR about *40%* below normal.
* Testes does **not** produce fructose.
* FSH level is high in post menopausal women.
* Fetal lung maturation depends on increased fetal **Cortisol** just before birth.
* LH is concerned with follicle maturation and ovulation.
* Testosterone is synthesized from **pregnanolone.**
* Metyrapone is used in treating **CAH** (Congenital Adrenal Hyperplasia).
* **Alloxan** causes diabetes.
* ADH acts on **Collecting tubules.**
* Adrenalin does not penetrate the cell membrane.
* TRH stimulated TSH and prolactin.
* Thyroxine has no role in response to **trauma.**
* HPL (Human placental lactogen) acts as GH for fetus.
* Chief metabolite of Estrogen in post menopusal women is sterone.
* Anabolic action on protein metabolism is mediated by **Testosterone.**
* Target Cellular organ for estrogen is nucleus.
* Menopausal hot flushes is due to **LH** surge.
* Increase in insulin receptor is seen in **starvation.**
* Male sex hormone is secreted mainly by **Interstitial cells** of Leydig.
* Development of male sex organ in fetal life depends on **testosterone** produced under the influence of HCG.
* Testosterone circulates in Combination with Gonadal steroid binding globulin.

* Estrogen increases the secretion and ciliary beating in fallopian tubes.
* Estrogen changes the cuboidal lining of vagina to stratified.
* Estrogen changes the break down of glycogen into lactate in vagina.
* Estrogen **initiates** breast development.
* Estrogen causes early **epiphyseal closure.**
* Estrogen causes water retention.
* Most important function of progesterone is to promote secretory changes in endometrium.
* Progesterone **completes** breast development by promoting alveolar and lobular development.
* Progesterone competes with aldosterone and thus causes Na & H2O excretion.
* **Progesterone** is the hormone for maintenance of pregnancy.
* Progesterone **inhibits** ovulation.
* Progesterone **decreases** membrane excitability by increasing resting membrane potential.
* Theca interna produces **estrogen** while Granulosa cells produce Progesterone.
* The hormone used for treating osteoporosis in old age — Testosterone.
* Aldosterone causes retention of Na+ & Cl-, H2O.
* Aldosterone acts on distal tubules in kidney, duct system of salivary glands, intestine.
* Aldosterone helps in maintaining excitability by preventing Hypokalaemia and Hyperpolarization.
* Glucocorticoids reduces cellular protein of all parts of the body **except liver.**
* Glucocorticoids **increase** Gluconeogenesis in liver.
* Glucocorticoids mobilize fatty acids from adipose tissues, thus increase plasma FFA.
* Glucocorticoids increase pepsin and gastric acid secretion.
* Glucocorticoids facilitate water insoluble lipid absorption while prevent calcium reabsorption (Because it is antagonistic to Vit. D).
* Glucocorticoids causes Eosinopenia, Lymphocytopenia.
* Miscible pool of calcium ion is the Calcium present in Periosteal space (1% of total).
* Largest endocrine gland in human —Thyroid.
* **Wolff Chalkoff effect** — Above a critical level, intrathyroidal I inhibits organic binding.

* Phenytoin, Salicylates compete with T3 & T4 for binding to TBG.
* Chronic hypothyroidism causes atherosclerosis.
* T4 causes breakdown of hyaluronic acid therapy increases urinary hexodamines.
* Thyroid hormone is necessary for conversion of β carotene to Vitamin A.
* Thyroid hormone decreases PO4 and calcium contentof body but increases Mg.
* Hypothyroidism causes constipation.
* Thyroid hormone may cause erythroid hyperplasia of Bone marrow.
* Extreme somnolence is a feature of hypothyroidism.
* Coupling reaction is inhibited by propylthiouracil, methimazole, carbimazole.
* Iodide trapping is inhibited by **thiocyanate,** perchlorate & nitrates.
* Inhibitors of insulin secretion — Epinephrine, insulin, starvation, hypoxia, vagotomy, serotonin.
* Stimulators of insulin secretion — Glucose, A.A., Ketones, ATP, AMP.
* Hormones derivd from cholesterol — Glucocorticoids, Mineralocorticoids, Estrogens, Progestins, Androgens, Calcitriol.
* Hormones requiring **cAMP** as second messenger — Ant. pit. hormones (except GH), ADH, PTH, Calcitonin, Glucagon.
* Hormones requiring Ca or phosphatidylinositol as 2nd messenger — ADH, TRH, LHRH, Angiotensin II, Acetylcholine specific protein.
* Hormones bound to **Globulins** in plasma — Hydrocortisone, Estrogen, Testosterone, T3,T4.
* Down regulation of receptors is seen with Insulin, Glucagon, GH, TRH, LH, FSH, Catecholamines.
* Acidophil cells of Anterior pituitary produce Basophil cells produces — GH, Prolactin (PRL) — FSH, LH, TSH, ACTH.
* Growth promoting action of GH is mediated through **Somatomedin-C** which is synthesized in Liver, Muscle, Kidney.
* **Somatomedin** causes depositition of chondroitin sulphate and collagen.
* GH can cause fatty liver and ketoacidosis by excesive mobilization of fat from adipose tissues.
* Anteriorior pituitory hormones with diabetogenic effect—GH, ACTH, TSH, PRL.
* GH enhances transport of aminoacids into **muscle** cells.
* Potent stimulus of GH secretion is **hypoglycemia** under acute condition while protein deficiency in chronic conditions.

* **Arginine** is the potent stimulus for GH secretion.
* Somatostatin is produced from **D cells** of Pancreas and Hypothalamus. It inhibits the secretion of GH,Insulin,Glucagon,TSH FSH,ACTH.
* In Laron dwarfs the GH levels are high. IGF-I is deficient.
* ADH is released from**Supraoptic nucleus** and is bound toneurophysinII while oxytocin from **Paraventricular nucleus** is bound to neurophysinI.
* Alcohol causes diuresis because it inhibits ADH secretion.
* Hypercalcemia may cause diuresis by inhibiting ADH secretion.
* In males FSH promotes spermatogenesis byenhancing the transport of **Testosterone** to seminiferous tubules and epidydmis by androgen binding protein synthesis from sertoli cells.
* LH stimulates progesterone synthesis from corpus luteum in females,testosterone synthesis from leydig cells from males.
* **Stein Leventhal syndrome** is characterized by polycystic ovary,raised LH\,increased androgen production.
* **Inhibin** inhibitsFSH release in males(from testis).
* TRH stimulates prolactin release.
* POMC(Pro-opio melanocortin)family includes-ACTH,MSH,LPH and endorphins.
* **Somatostatin** inhibits secretion of gastrin, secretin, VIP and GIP
* **Secretin** is a polypeptide with 27 aminoacids and a fall of pH below 4.5 causes prompt increase in its secretion
* **Insulin** was first discovered by Banting and Best in 1921 extracted from pancreas. Crystallized insulin was prepared by Abel in 1926. Detailed amino acid structure by elucidated by Sanger in 1952. Proinsulin was discovered by Steiner in 1967. Three dimensional structure was given by Dorothy Hodgkin in 1969
* F-cells (P-cells) in pancreas secrete pancreatic polypeptide. Alpha cells secrete glucagon, Beta cells insulin and delta cells- gastrin and somatostatin.
* Thyroid hormones have prominent effects on bone resorption and formation
* Insulin has prominent effect on bone formation
* OCP's or excessive estrogens increases thyroxine binding globulin whereas prednisolone, excessive androgens, phenytoin decreases TBG
* **Drug of choice** in diabetes insipidus is desmopressin.
* Virilization in Stein Levinthal syndrome is due to increased secretion of ovarian androgens.
* Triiodothyronine is **most rapidly acting** thyroid preparation.

* Steroids are used to stop fibrosis.
* Medical adrenalectomy is produced by aminoglulethimide.
* Insulin can be given I/V is crystalline zinc insulin.
* Chlorpropamide enhance the action of ADH on distal nephron.
* Drugs useful in Rx of SIADH—Demeclocycline (a tetracycline derivative)
* Demeclocycline inhibits the action of ADH on the collecting duct.
* **Drugs causing Nephrogenic diabetes insipidus**
    * Lithium
    * Demeclocycline
* One of the complications due to insulin—Presbyopia.
* Chlorpropamide causes facial flushing after ingestion of alcohol.
* Chromium deficiency causes insulin resistance.
* **Drugs also useful in treatment of Diabetes insipidus**
    * Clofibrate—increase vasopressin secretion
* Glucogon exerts its effect on glucose output via a protein kinase that inhibits glycogen synthesis, facilities glycogenolysis, and inhibits conversion of phosphoenol pyruvate to pyruvate.
* Drugs that inhibit insulin secretion—Diazoxide, Thiazide, diuretics.
* Biguanides do not affect insulin secretion but increase glucose utilisation. They increase anaerobic glycolysis within the cells. They also decrease glucose absorption from the gastrointestinal tract.
* Metyrapone inhibits Adrenal 11β-Hydroxylase.
* Desmopressin is used in oesophageal varices, diabetes insipidus, nocturnal enuresis, mild to moderate hemophilia, hemophilia type A, von Willebrand type I and is contraindicated in vascular disease, CAD, chr. nephritis and von Willebrand's type II B.
* Effects of desmopressin are increased by carbamazepine and chlorpropamide.
* Glucagon receptors are on cell membrane.
* Syndrome of inappropiate ADH secretion (**SIADH**) is caused by Chlorpropamide.
* Insulinoma is diagnosed by Tolbutamide.
* **Mifepristone** is used for termination of pregnancy.
* Estrogen treatment is associated with Hepatocellular adenoma.
* Endocrine manifestations as a side effect are caused by Ketoconazole.
* **Most common** side effect of prolonged use of steroids is affective disorders.

* Androgen, estrogen and progesterone act on protein regulation through nuclear receptor except GnRH.
* Diabetes insipidus—**Vasopressin, Desmopressin (DDAVP)**
* Thyrotoxicosis patients preparing for thyroidectomy—**Propylthiouracil and Iodine (preopmethod of choice)**
* Thyrotoxicosis in pregnancy—**Propranolol**
* Hypoparathyroid testing—calciferol
* Adrenal crisis—**Hydrocortisone sodium succinate.**
* Addison's disease—**Hydrocortisone**
* Hypercalcemia due to hypervitaminosis D—**Steroids**
* **Glucogonomas** arise from the α-cells of the pancreatic islets
* Craniopharyngiomas are tumors that arise from remnants of Rathke's pouch.
* The 21-hydroxylase deficiency is most commonly found form of the adrenogenital syndrome.
* The thyroid cancer most frequently metastasises to lymph nodes is papillary.
* Multiple endocrine neoplasia (MEN) are familial disorders with autosomal dominant mode of transmission.
* MEN II syndrome is characterized by the occurrence of medullary carcinoma thyroid, pheochromocytomas and parathyroid hyperplasia.
* Affection of terminal ileum in Crohn's disease is called as ***back wash ileitis."***
* Ulcerative colitis is primarily a disease of mucosa.
* Thyroid appearance of renal tubules is considered **pathognomonic** of chronic pyelonephritis.
* One of the causes of Hypercalcemia — Addison's disease.
* HPA axis starts working during **20th week** of Intrauterine life.
* Synthesis of Thyroglobulin starts in **8th week** of intrauterine life.
* In Diabetes insipidus, urinary S.G. is **1.001—1.005** but serum osmolality is normmal.
* In diabetes mellitus (DM), poor prognostic factors are proteinuria within **15 years** of DM, and age **10-20 years.**
* Half life of insulin is **4-7 minutes** irrespective of dose injected.
* The **insulin-to-glucagon ratio** determines the rate of ketogenesis by the liver.
* The occurrence of hyperglycaemic ketoacidosis or hyperglycemmic hyperosmolar coma is diagnostic of diabetes mellitus.

* **Insulin allergy** occurs 1 to 4 weeks after insulin is started.
* **Insulin resistance** is present in patient requiring over 200 IU insulin daily provided there is no infection, obesity or other medical or endocrinal disorders requiring increased insulin need.
* The oat cell carcinoma of the bronchus is the most common nonendocrine tumour secreting ACTH.
* **Sheehan's syndrome** is usually caused by infarction of the anterior pituitary (Post partum infarction).
* Pseudohypoparathyroidism is a rare genetic disorder inherited as an x-linked dominant trait.
* Patient with Turner's syndrome is called chromatin negative.
* The **somatostatinoma** arises from the D cells of the islets of pancreas.
* **Reftoff's syndrome** results from apparent resistance of the peripheral tissue to the action of thyroid hormone.
* SIADH results from the continued secretion of ADH.
* Craniopharyngiomas are tumors arising from remnant of Rathke's pouch.
* The 21 hydroxylase deficiency is the most commonly found form of the adrenogenital syndrome.
* Excessive sweating may be the **most reliable** clinical sign of activity of gigantism disease.
* The most important cause of high serum prolactin is a pituitary tumour.
* Inappropriate secretion of ADH is most commonly caused by oat cell bronchogenic carcinoma.
* Thyrotoxicosis associated with ocular signs or ocular disturbances and with a diffuse goitre is called Grave's disease.
* **Ellsworth-Howard test** (phosphaturia after administration of I/V 200 units of parathyroid hormone) is used to differentiate true hypoparathyroidism (responds to parathyroid extract) and, pseudohypoparathyroidism (does not respond).
* Prolonged hypocalcemia due to recalcification of the hungry skeleton may require large amounts of calcium and vitamin D.
* The most **reliable test** for phaeochromocytoma associated with paroxysmal hypertension is direct assay of epinephrine and norepinephrine in the blood & urine during or following an attack.
* The most common primary developmental abnormality causing hypogonadism is Klinefelter's syndrome.
* Bilateral atrophy of the first interosseous muscles of the hand is characteristic of diabetic neuropathy (ankle jerk is often absent but knee jerk may be retained).

* Medications that may impair glucose tolerance include diuretics, contraceptive drugs, glucocorticoids, nicotinic acid and phenytoin.
* The signs and symptoms of **pituitary apoplexy** depend on the patient's underlying endocrine status, the amount of damage or compromise to contiguous brain structures, and the severity and pattern of hormonal dropout.
* States of normal total body sodium and excesss free water are usually the result of inappropriate secretion or action of ADH as a result of tumors, leakage of ADH, or drug effects.
* **Hypermagnesemia** is **rare** unless renal function is impaired.
* Severe hypophosphatemia is often accompanied by other metabolic abnormalities (hypokalemia, hypocalcemia hypomagnesemia).
* **Diabetic ketoacidosis** (DKA) is caused by an insulin deficiency by hyperglycemia and ketonemia.
* Consider the diagnosis of hypoglycemia in any person who has altered mental function.
* Type I diabetics without a normal secretory response of glucagon and epinephrine are at increased risk for hypoglycemia.
* **Nonketotic hyperosmolar coma** (NKHC) is characterized by profound hyperglycemia without significant ketosis. The mainstay of treatment is fluids.
* **Alcoholic ketoacidosis** (AKA) is characterized by significant ketoacidosis and serum glucose levels that can vary from mild hyperglycemia to frank hypoglycemia.
* Adrenal insufficiency results from a primary adrenal disorder or secondary to a lack of ACTH. The most common cause is chronic steroid therapy with hypothalamic-pituitary-adrenal axis suppression.
* The Cushing syndrome may result from pituitary (**most common**) or ectopic sources of ACTH, or from primary adrenal hypercortisolemia.
* Management of pheochromocytomas involves alpha adrenergic blockade followed by beta adrenergic blockade; doses must be individually tailored.
* Surgical resection of pheochromocytomas should be preceded by **at least weeks of stabilization** of the blood pressure, heart rate, and plasma volume.
* **Somatostatin** (GHRIH) produces ↓ GH and ↓ in plasma-gastrin, glucagon, insulin and platelet stickiness.
* Although insulin antibodies of the IgG type are present in almost every diabetic individual within the first 60 days of insulin therapy, they are almost never present in untreated individuals.

* **HbAIC** make up about 5 to 8% of Hb of persons without diabetes, whereas in persons with poorly controlled diabetes it accounts for an average of 10 to 24% of Hb.
* The rate of **glycosylated Hb** (HbAIC) formation is dependent on the average plasma glucose level during the
* Phenformin may cause lactic acidosis.lifespan of the red blood cell (nearly 120 days).
* Common cause of galactorrhea-amonorrhea syndrome is a prolactin-secreting tumor of primary gland.
* Neonatal tetany is probably due to the high phosphate content of milk and relative hypoparathyroidism.
* Obesity is not common in hypothyroidism.
* Hashimoto's thyroiditis often leads to hypothyroidism.
* Diabetes mellitus may appear with the menopause.
* Hypoglycaemia is a recognised feature of primary hepatoma.
* Coincident acidosis usually **prevents** tentany.
* E.S.R. level is increased in cretinism.
* When CCF sets in bradycardia of myxoedema gives way to tachycardia.
* **Hirsutism** is noted in Cushing's syndrome.
* Treatment is **life long** in myxoedema.
* Pituitary dwarfs have intelligence.
* **Insulin resistant diabetes** shall be controlled by 200 Units insulin + steroids.
* Insulin resistant diabetics is also called pseudotabes.
* Thyrotoxicosis causes palmar erythema.
* **Adrenal crisis** may be precipitated by thyroid therapy of pituitary myxoedema.
* Nervousness is a common finding in adult hypothyroidism.
* Tetany can produce laryngeal stridor is infants.
* **'Apathetic' hyperthyroidism** is commoner in the aged.
* Diabetic glomerulosclerosis is the specific pathological lesion in diabetic nephropathy.
* Hashimoto's disease shows high titre of thyroid antibodies.
* Acromegaly patient will have hypertension as one of clinical signs.
* Hypopituitarism resulting from postpartum necrosis of pituitary is called **Sheehan's syndrome.**

Non-insulin secreting adenoma, hyperacidity and peptic ulcer refers to **Zollinger Ellison syndrome.**

* Tetany is relieved by administration of calcium gluconate.
* Tetany can occur from hyperventilation.
* Acromegaly will come with manifestation of polyarthropathy.
* Pretibial myxoedema is a manifestation of thyrotoxicosis.
* Hypoglycaemia is a recognised feature of primary hepatoma.
* Keto steroid excretion in urine is increased in phaeohromocytoma.
* Coincident acidosis usually prevents tetany.
* In primry myxoedema TSH level in blood is increased.
* Eosinophil adenoma of pituitary gives rise to acromegaly.
* E.S.R. level is increased in cretinism
* Myxoedema patient can present with psychotic manifestations.
* The onset of ketoacidotic coma is quick.
* Duration of Lente insulin is 24 hours.
* When CCF sets in, bradycardia of myxoedema gives way to tachycardia.
* **Hirsutism** is noted in Cushing's syndrome.
* PBI andT4 are decreased in myxoedema.
* Addison's disease is associated with hyponatremia and Hypokalemia.
* In pregnancy, diabetes should be controlled by insulin and diet.
* Increased TSH levels in blood indicate primary type of myxoedema.
* Treatment is **life long** in myxoedema.
* Blood sugar is **normal** in renal glycosuria.
* Rice diet is **contraindicated** in diabetes.
* Diabetics often suffer from tuberculosis.
* Fine tremors, tachycardia and warm moist hands suggest Thyrotoxicosis.
* Reactive hyperglycemia may be a feature in some diabetic patients.
* Pituitary inturn is controlled by Hypothalamus.
* Moniliasis is common in diabetes mellitus.
* **Carpo-pedal spasm** is commonly due to deficiency of parathormone.
* Relaxation of tendon jerk is slow in myxoedema endocrine disease.
* Diabetes is generally regulated during pregnancy with insulin.
* The adrenal gland disorder producing hypertension without hyperglycemia is conn's syndrome.
* Plain insulin is **the drug of choice** in diabetic ketoacidosis.
* Hypoglycaemia is more dangerous than hyperglycaemia.
* The endocrinal disease that produces tetany is hypoparathyroidism.
* Long standing diabetes mellitus is associated with proteinuria and hypertension.

* Thyrotoxicosis causes palmar erythema.
* Organic psychoses with paranoid delusions may occur in myxoedema.
* Obesity is not common in hypothyroidism.
* Nervousness is a common finding in adult hypothyroidism
* Glucose intolerance is seen in many patients with familial type IV, but hypertriglyceridemia of this pattern occurs in diabetes.
* Chlorpropamide is **not metabolized** and is excreted almost completely in the urine.
* Tolbutamide is precipitated by acidifying the urine. Alcohol intolerance has been seen with sulfonylurea administration.
* In hypersmolar hyperglycemic non-ketotic coma, the blood glucose level is around **55 mmol/l.**
* **Most common** presentation of primary hyperparathyroidism is subtle neurological and Psychiatric symptoms.
* Treatment of **Hypercalcemia** is Plicamycin, Bisdionate and gallium nitrate.
* Central Diabetes Insipidus is characterised by low plasma and low urine osmolality.
* To monitor therapy response in hypothyroidism, best is TSH.
* Adenomas in Parathyroid are most often located in inferior parathyroid.
* The residual form of **pheochromocytoma** is treated by MIBG.
* Immunosupressed diabetics in ketoacidosis appear to be particularly susceptible to zygomycosis.
* A high plasma calcitonin level causes increased formation of 24-25 dihydroxy cholecalciferol.
* Albuminuria symptom excludes hyperaldosteronism.
* Congenital malformation of fetus is DM diagnosed by HbA1AC.
* In ectopic ACTH due to small Ca lung, seen is Hypokalemic alkalosis.
* Paradoxical GH increases with administration of TSH in Acromegaly, Malnutrition and Anorexia nervosa.
* **Adrenomedullary triad** of excessive amounts of adrenomedullary catecholeamines consists of tachycardia, vasoconstriction and sweating.
* Spontaneous testicular descent does not occur after the age of 1 year.
* **Isosexual precocity** refers to an abnormally early onset (girtls **<8 years** of age, boys <9 years of age) of sexual characteristics appropriate to the child's sex, with eventual attainment of full sexual maturation and premature closure of epiphyses.

* Patients with GH deficiency have a subnormal rate of growth (**<4.0 cm/ year** after the age of 4-5 years).
* The **most common** cause of sporadic goiter is lymphocytic thyroiditis.
* The most common cause of thyroid disease in children & adolescents is lymphocytic thyroiditis (Hashimoto thyroiditis or Autoimmune thyroiditis)
* In infants, Cushing syndrome is **most often** caused by a functioning **enocortical** tumour.
* The **most common** site of origin of phaeochromocytoma is the adrenal medulla.
* The **most common** endocrine-metabolic disease in childhood is Insulin-dependent diabetes mellitus (IDDM) type I
* The **most commonly** used thyroid imaging technique in children is Technetium 99m (99mTc) scanning.
* The **most common** cause of GH deficiency is idiopathic & in majority of cases the defect is in hypothalamus.
* The **most common** cause of primary ovarian failure is Turner syndrome.
* The **most common** causes of adrenocortical insufficiency in infancy are the salt-losing forms of congenital adrenal hyperplasia.
* The **most common** infection associated with calcifications within the adrenal is tuberculosis & patient usually has clinical manifestations of Addison's disease.
* The most common causes of instability or "brittleness" in diabetic children are the Somogyi & Dawn phenomena together.A
* The **most common** of the aminoacid disorders is phenyketonuria (PKU)
* The **most common** inborn error of metabolism of methionine is homocystinemia type I or classic homocystinuria.

INVESTIGATIONS

* T3 as measured by radio-immuneo-assay (RIA) is particularly useful indiagnosing hyperthyroidism.
* Measurement of free T4 is usually not necessary for appropriate diagnosis
* TSH measurement by RIA is valuable in diagnosis of primary hypothyroidism
* Uses of 99m Tc scanning—for identificaiton of 'cold' nodules (areas of uptake of radionuclide), for localization of ectopic thyroid tissue or absence of thyroid tissue.

* Ultrasound of thyroid—useful in characterization of cystic lesions of the thyroid.
* T3 resin uptake—an indirect measure of the patients thyroid binding protein (T3 resin uptake is in hyperthyroidism & in hypothyroidism)
* Presence of thyrotropin-binding inhibition immunoglobulin (TB II) & Thyroid-stimulating immunoglobulins (TSI) correlates with disease activity in hyperthyroidism (Graves disease) in childhood.
* Radioactive iodine uptake is rarely performed in children as a diagnostic test (I^{123} is preferred over I^{131}).
* Absence of 99m Tc uptake indicates thyroid agensis & 99 m Tc uptake in a normally positioned gland implies an enzymatic defect in thyroid hormone production.
* A reliable index of long-term glycermic control in diabetics is provided by measurement of glycosylated haemoglobin.
* The most direct & specific test for phaeochroneocytoma is the demonstration of basal plasma levels or excretion of catechlomines.
* Congenital hypothyroidsm—serum total T4, T3 resin uptake & serum TSH; localization of 99m Tc uptake (ectopic gland).
* Juvenile (acquired hypothyroidism)—serum total T4, T3 resin uptake & serum. TSH; circulating thyroid autoantibodies (autoimmune basis).
* Graves disease (thyrotoxicosis)—serum total T4 & Total T3, T4 with I131 uptake (due to surreptitious overdosing with thyroid hormone).
* Neonatal graves disease—thyroid hormone levels & TSH
* Thyroiditis—titers of thyroid autoantibodies (antithyroglobulin & antimicrosomal antibodies); normal serum T4 & TSH or normal T4 with TSH (compensated hypothyridism) or T4 levels with TSH (hypothyroidism)
* Congenital adrenal hyperplasia (adrenogenital syndrome)—
* Classical salt-wasting 21-hydroxylase deficiency—measurement of markedly levels of serum 17 hydroxyprogesterone
* Simple virilizing 21-hydroxylase deficiency—serum 17 - hydroxyprogesterone
* Nonclassical 21-hydroxylase deficiency (acquired or late - onset) — excessive of 17-hydroxy-progesterone after ACTH stimulation.
* 11- Hydroxylase deficiency —serum 11 - deoxycortisol & deoxycortisol & deoxycorticosterone or their tetrahydro-metabolites in urine.
* Primary adrenal insufficiency (adrenocortical insufficiency)— Hyponatremia, hyperkalemia, mild metabolic; serum cortisol level
* Cushing syndrome—serum cortisol, absence of normal diurnal variation, overnight dexamethasone suppression test.

* Phaeochromocytoma—↑ epinephrine, norepinephrine or ↑ urinary VMA.
* Goiter is almost always present in the congenitally hyperthyroid infant.
* Graves' disease is the only disease known to be caused by an antibody which stimulates endocrine cell.
* Type I diabetes IDDM is associated with HLA antigens (DR3, DR4 & B8), circulating antibodies to cytoplasmic & cell surface components of islet cells, & hytoplastic infiltration of islets.
* Rapid infusion of bicarbonate is contraindicated in while correcting acidosis in diabetic ketoacidosis (becasuse it may cause deterioration of neurologic function & CSF pH.
* The **first symptom** of congenital hypothyroidism is prolonged neonatal jaundice.
* The total dose of insulin for a child may be based upon age or size rather than upon the degress of hyperglycemia or glycosuria.
* Children with Down's syndrome have an incidence of hypothyroidism & hyperthyroidism
* The drug of choice for diabetes insipidus is Desmopressin.
* Children with diabetes insipidus do not perspire (their skin in dry & plate)
* Corticosteroids are contraindicated in the treatment of Reye syndrome because of their catabolic effects.
* A child is considered to have impaired glucose tolerange (IGT) if the fasting plasma glucose concentration <140 mg/dl but the 2-hour value exceeds 140 mg/dl.
* Cortiocosteriods are used in treatment of Idiopathic thrombocytopenic purpura.
* Severe hyperglycaemia as a complication of intravenous alimentation is seen in the early stages of treatment in low birth weight infants.
* Primary adrenal insufficuency in the newborn may be due to overwhelming sepsis.
* A hypothyroid child exhibits decreased sweating.
* Diabetes insipidus in association with diabetes mellitus, optic atrophy and sensorineural deafness is characteristic of Wolfram syndrome.
* Acquired hypothyroidim (Juvenile hypothyroidism) most often results from Lymphocytic thyroiditis (Hashimoto or autoimmune thyroiditis)
* The earliest sign in children with Graves' disease is emotional disturbance with motor hyperactivity.
* In infants, Cushing's syndrome is most often caused by functioning adrenocortical tumour.

* An index of lonterm hyperglycaemic control is determined by measurement of **Glycosated haemoglobin**.
* **Klinefelter's syndrome** is associated with advanced maternal age.
* Fructose is not used for IV infusion as it causes lactic acidosis
* Chromophobe adenomas occur most commonly in female patients between the age of 20 and 50.
* The most common kind of pituitary tumours are chromophobe adenomas.
* Papillary carcinoma is the most common of the malignant tumours of the thyrod (2/3rd of all thyroid carcinomas).
* Diarrhoea is the most common complaint in medullary carcinoma of thyroid.
* Hashimoto's disease or chronic lymphocytic thyroditis, is the most common form of chronic thyroditis.
* The commonest site of thyroglossal cyst is beneath the hyoid.
* The most common cause of hypoparathyroidism is surgical removal.
* The most common cause of hypercalcaemia of malignant disease is osseous metastasis.
* Parathyroid adenomata most commonly are made up of chief cells.
* The most common type of congenital adrenal hyperplasia is due to deficiency of 21-hydroxylase.
* 'Focal calcification' is most commonly seen in nodular goitre.
* Elevated plasma bound iodoalbumin is often seen in Thyroid cancer.
* The commonest symptom and sign of hyperparathyroidism are Renal colic and Renal stone.
* The commonest cause of hypercalcaemia found in clinical practice is carcinoma breast with bone metastasis while receiving oestrogen therapy.
* The most common cause of adrenal insufficiency is use of cortisone.
* Cushing's syndrome is most commonly seen in adrenal hyperplasia.
* The commonest cause for Addison's disease is due to tuberculous infection.
* A single adenoma is the commonest finding in primary hyperparathyroidism.
* The most common presentation of asymptomatic hyperparathyroidism cases is the detection of unsuspected and asymptomatic hypercalcaemia by routine hiochemical screening.
* Cushing's syndrome is the commonest form of endogenous hypercorticism accounting for up to 2/3rds of all cases.
* **Most common** cause of adrenal crisis – Sudden withdrawai of steroids.

* **Most common** cause of Hyper calcemia in adults – Hyper parathyroidism
* **Most common** cause of pancreatic calcification – Alcoholism.
* **Most common** type of hormone secreted ectopically is – Peptide/ protein hormone.
* **Most common** part of endocrine system involved in sarcoidosis – Hypothalamic pituitary axis (Diabetes insipius)
* **Most common symptom** of medullary Ca Thyroid is Diarrhoea.
* Patients with MEN syndrome have defect in **Chromosome-10.**
* **Most common** presenting feature in thyroid cancer is Goitre.
* **Most common** cause of **solitary thyroid nodule** is follicular adenoma.
* **Most common** pathalogy of pancreas in MEN-1 is **Carcinoma.**
* **Most common** pathalogy in MEN-IIA is **Medullary CA of thyroid.**
* Most common symptom of prolactinoma in male is Decreased Libido.
* Most common pituitary adenoma is Sparsely Granulated Prolactinoma.
* Most common site of primary cancer which gives rise to secondary in the adrenal gland is lung.
* Most common cause of hyperpituitarism is Adenoma.
* Most common presentation of adrenal cortical carcinoma is Cushing's syndrome.
* Hypopituitarism should be first treated with corticosteroids.
* The thyroid gland is developed from the median bud of the pharynx (the thyroglossal duct).
* Paired superior thyroid arteries arise from the external carotid arteries whereas Paired inferior thyroid arteries arise from the thyrocervical trunks of the subclavian arteries.
* A fifth artery, **the thyroid ima**, is sometimes present and arises from the arch of aorta and enters the thyroid in midline.
* Superior thyroid vein & middle thyroid veins join the internal jugular vein whereas inferior thyroid veins join the brachiocephalic (innominate) vein.
* The upper parathyroids arise embryologically from the fourth branchial pouch along with the analyge of the thyroid. The lower parathyroids arise from the third branchial pouch along with the thymus and descend with the thymus.
* Upper pair of parathyroids are more **constant** in position than the lower pair.
* Left adrenal gland is little larger than the right.

* Right side adrenal vein in short and enters the IVC, whereas left adrenal vein empties into left renal vein.
* Adrenal cortex has **no known innervation.**
* **D-cells** secrete Somatostatin
* Parathyroid tetany, due to hypocalcaemia, is a rare complication of subtotal thyroidectomy (< 1%), but a more common complication of total thyroidectomy.
* The most important complication of thyroid adenoma is **malignant transformation.**
* In secondary thyrotoxicosis the goitre is nodular and the hyperthyroidism is not severe and eye signs other than lid lag and lid spasm are very rare.
* Pregnancy may lead to an exacerbation of a variety of autoimmune diseases in the postpartum period **(postpartum hyperthyroidism)**.
* Papillary carcinoma usually presents as an asymptomatic nodule within the thyroid gland or as an enlargement of the regional lymph nodes.
* **Riedel's thyroiditis** is thought by some to be a terminal stage of Hashimoto's disease or granulomatous thyroiditis.
* It is now felt that the so-called lateral aberrant thyroid almost always represents papillary – follicular carcinoma that has metastasized from a primary thyroid cancer and has replaced a lymph node with tumor.
* The **first symptom** of hypoparathyroidism are tingling and numbness in the face, fingers and toes.
* Sudden stoppage of long continued cortisone treatment results in rebound cortical deficiency.
* Most patients with multinodular goitre are asymptotic and do not require operation (indicated on cosmetic grounds).
* The term **myxoedema** should be used only for the very advanced form of adult hypothyroidism.
* Endemic cretinism is often goitrous and is usually due to iodine deficiency.
* In many cases of toxic nodular goitre, the nodules are inactive, and it is internodular thyroid tissue that is overactive.
* Neonatal thyrotoxicosis occurs in babies born to hyperthyroid mothers or to euthyroid mothers who have had thyrotoxicosis.
* Almost all cases of hyperplasia are of the **chief cell type**.
* A **thyroglossal cyst** is mostly seen in teenagers.
* Iodine is lethal to proliferating cells in the depth of wound and delays normal wound healing.

* Papillary carcinoma may contain localised deposits of calcium arranged in concentric layers (**psammoma bodies**).
* Papillary carcinoma has frequently followed accidental irradiation of the thyroid in childhood.
* Follicular carcinoma incidence is high in endemic goitrous areas (possibly due to TSH stimulation).
* De Quervain's thyroiditis is due to a virus infection.
* **In de Quervain's thyroiditis** there is - ESR, absent tyroid antibodies, - T4 and 123 I uptake.
* The **best method** to localise parathyroid gland is hyperparathyroidism is to do selective angiography of the inferior tyroid artery.
* The **commonest** lesion which fails to takeup 75 Se-selenomethionine but can take up 1131 is nodular goitre.
* When adrenal insufficiency is suspected, the most useful test is 24 hours urinary sodium (second is ACTH stimulation test).
* Distinction between follicular adenoma and follicular carcinoma is usually only possible onthe basis of histological evidence of invasion through the capsule or into the blood vessels.
* A discrete thyroid swelling in a teenager of either sex must be provisionally diagnosed as carcinoma.
* The **most significant** symptoms of thyrotoxicosis are loss of weight inspite of a good appeitite, a recent preference for cold, and palpitations.
* The **most significant** signs of thyrotoxicosis are excitability of patient, presence of goire, exophthalmos and tachycardia or cardiac arrhythmia.
* Papillary carcinoma is the **most slowly growing** malignant tumours of thyroid.
* Women under treatment with antityroid drugs may give birth to a hypothyroid infant.
* Antithyroid drugs **cannot cure** a toxic nodule.
* **Sporadic cretinism** is due to complete or near complete failure of thyroid development (partial failure causes juvenile myxoedema).
* In **Sheehan's syndrome**, after delivery, there is failure of lactation.
* Asymptomatic hypocalcaemia is seen in hypoproteinaemia (due to free ionised calcium level is normal in blood).
* Hyperthyroidism (Thyrotoxicosis factitia) may be induced by taking l-thyroxine but only if the dosage exceeds thenormal requirements of 0.2 to 0.3 mg a day.
* Exophthalmos is nearly always absent in secondary thyrotoxicosis.

* Thyroglossal fistula is **never** congenital.
* An ectopic thyroid is usually mistaken for sublingual dermoid.
* Absent carotid pulse in thyroid swelling suggests malignancy.
* Repeated occurrence of urinary calculi suggests hyperparathyroidism.
* Most important pre and post operative measure to be taken before adrenalectomy is giving corticosteroid.
* Fine needle aspiration cytology (FNAC) cannot distinguish between a benign follicular adenoma and follicular carcinoma.
* T_3 is metabolically more active than T_4
* Half life of T_3 is 3 days
* **Lingual-thyroid** is a rounded swelling **at back of tongue at foramen caecum** and it may represent the only thyroid gland of body.
* **Mitotane** is the only chemotherapeutic agent of proved value in Adrenal carcinoma.
* **Phaeochromocytoma**
* Also known as **chromaffin tumor**, as it arises from chromaffin cells
* Extra adrenal tumors have higher incidence of malignancy
* β-blockers should never be administered without prior alpha adrenergic blockage in Pheochromocytoma.
* Most common metabolic abnormality which may develop after operation in a patient of pheochromocytoma is **Hypoglycemia.**
* Most common site of metastases of malignant pheochromocytoma is bone and lung.
* Treatment of pheochromocytoma in Early pregnancy is the surgical removal as soon as the diagnosis is confirmed, provided that the patient is prepared with phenoxybenzamine preoperatively.
* Malignant pheochromocytomas are more common in **children** and in **extra-adrenal tumors.**
* First biochemical abnormality detected in MEN-1 is **Hyperparathyroidism.** Most common manifestation is Hypercalcemia.
* Second most common expression of MEN-1 is neoplasia of the **Pancreatic islet cells** (Most common is **parathyroid hyperplasia).**
* **First abnormality** detected in MEN-II Medullary CA of thyroid.
* The pheochromocytomas are **nearly always** limited to the adrenal medulla, nearly always **benign** and nearly **always Bilateral.**
* Non endocrine manifestations of **MEN IIB.**
    * "Marfanoid body habitus"
    * Mucosal neuroma ('Bumpy Lips')
    * Multiple mucocutaneous ganglioneuromas of GIT.

* Most consistently observed risk factor for Ca pancreas is smoking.
* Characteristic finding suggesting diagnosis of CA pancreas is a **constriction** of, both the pancreatic and bile ducts in the head of the gland. So this is called **double-duck sign.**
* About 20% of tumors of the head of pancreas are resectable at the time of operation.
* **Triad** of somatostatinoma includes : Diabetes mellitus (mild); Steatorrhoea and Cholelithiasis
* Glucagoma arises from alpha-cells (more precisely $\alpha 2$ cells) of pancreatic islets.
* The hall marks of the glucagonoma syndrome are **mild diabetes and severe dermatitis**.
* In thyroid malignancy, due to involvement of artery in malignant process, carotid pulsation is not felt. It is **Berry's sign.**

NAMED SIGNS

Thyrotoxicosis:

* **Boston's Sign**
  — Jerking of the lagging lid on elevation of the eye balls.
* **Dalrymple's Sign**
  — Widened palpebral fissure due to exophthalmos.
* **Guttman's Sign**
  — Bruit heard over thyroid on auscultation.
* **Jellinek's Sign** (Hyperthyroidism)
  — Brownish pigmentation of eyelids especially the upper.
* **Marie Sign**
  — Presence of tremors of extremities.
* **Grave's sign**
  — Failure to close the eyelids fully in sleep.
* **Mean's Sign**
  — Global lag during elevation of the eye ball
* **Von Graefe's Sign**
  (*Lid lag sign*)
  — Upper lid lags behind the globe as the gaze is lowered suddenly, momentarily unmasking the rim of sclera above the cornea.

Grave's Disease:

* **Backer's Sign**
  — increased pulsation in the retinal arteries.
* **Cowen's Sign**
  — Jerky consensual pupillary reaction.
* **Enroth's Sign**
  — Edema of the eyelids, especially of the upper lid near the supraorbital margin.
* **Griffith's Sign**
  — Lagging of the lower lid on upward gaze.
* **Knie's Sign**
  — unequal pupillary dilatation.
* **Rosenbach's Sign**
  — Fine rapid tremors of the upper lids, when the eyelids are gently closed.
* **Stellwag's Sign**
  — Infrequent & incomplete blinking of eyelids.
* **Wilder's Sign (early stages)**
  — Slight twitch of the eyeball, when it changes its movement from adduction to abduction or vice versa.

Exophthalmic goitre:

* **Abadie's Sign**
  — Spasm of levator palpebrae superioris muscle
* **Gifford's Sign**
  — Inability to evert the upper lid.
* **Mobius Sign**
  — Absence of convergence of eyes
* **Pemberton's Sign** - *Retrosternal goitre*
  — Patient is asked to elevate the arms, then there is engorgement of the face (due to pressure on great veins in the neck)
* **Berry's Sign** - Ca. Thyroid
  — On palpation absence of carotid pulsation in the neck.
* **Waltman's Sign** - *Myxoedema*
  — Slowing of deep reflexes especially ankle jerk.

Hypoparathyroidism (Latent tetany):

* **Chvostek's Sign** (hypocalcemic tetany)

— On tapping the trunk of facial nerve anterior to external auditory meatus produces drawing of mouth towards that side (due to spasm)

* **Escherich's Sign**

— Tapping of the skin at the ankle of mouth causes protrusion of lips.

* **Hochsinger's Sign** (hypocalcemic tetany)

— Closure of the hand occurs on application of the pressure to the inner aspect of biceps muscle.

* **Kashida's thermic Sign** (tetany)

— Development of hyperaesthesia and spasm following the application or either hot or cold irritants.

* **Peroneal Sign**

— Dorsal flexion and abduction of foot when the peroneal nerve is tapped just below the head of fibula, while the knee is slightly flexed.

* **Schultze's Sign**

— Tapping of tongue causes its depression with a concave dorsum.

* **Trousseau's Sign**

— Carpopedal spasm, elicited when the upper arm is com pressed by a tourniquet or a blood pressure cuff.

* **Knuckle-Dimple Sign**

(pseudohypoparathyroidism)

— On asking the patient make a fist, shortening of the 1st, 4th and 5th metacarpal bones is seen.

* **Flush-Tank Sign:** (Seen in) *Hydronephrosis*...passage of a large amount of urine and the coincident temporary disappearance of the lumbar swelling.
* **Gilbert's Sign:** (Seen in) Hepatic cirrhosis...more urine is se- creted during fasting than during digestion
* **Thornton's Sign:** (Seen in) *Nephrolithiasis*...Severe colicky pain is felt in the region of the flanks.

NAMED SYNDROMES

* **Klinefelter's syndrome**:

Karyotype:

47, XXY (Classical form)

46 XY/47 XXY (mosaicism)

Results from at least two X-chromosomes and Y chromosomes due to non-disjunction or malagregation of the sex chromosome during paternal or maternal meiosis.

— Small firm testess, azoospermia, gynaecomastia and elevated levels of plasma gonadotropins in men with two or more X chromosomes.

* Increased height due to increase in the length of legs, weak growth of facial hair, female distribution of fat and sexual hair, sterility low plasma testosterone levels, subnormal libido.

* Mild mental retardation and behavioural disturbances.

* **Turner's Syndrome**

(Gonadal dysgenesis)

Results from for chromosomal anomaly with 45 XO (only single X chromosome)

— Short stature, sheild shaped chest, valgus of elbows. Lymphedema of hands and feet, webbing of the neck, low hair line, redundant skin folds on the back of the neck. Primary amenorrhea, sexual infantilism, and bilaternal streak gonads in phenotypic women with sex chromatin negative.

* **Cushing syndrome:**

* *Excessive glucocorticoids* (due to adrenal hyperplasia and neoplasia)

— Moon facies, buffalo hump, protuberant abdomen, hirsutism, wasting of limbs, retarded growth, weakness, osteoporosis, amenorrhoea & glycosuria. Skin with acne, purplish striae and ecchymotic patches.

* **Cushing syndrome medicamentosa:**

— Excessive intake of corticosteroids (for a prolonged period)

* **Ectopic ACTH syndrome:**
  — *Excessive production of ACTH from, nonendocrine tissues* (ca. lung, thymomma, bronchial carcinoids and medullary ca. of thyroid) as Cushsing's Syndrome.
* **Harris syndrome:**
  Hyperinsulinism (functional islet cell tumours and pancreatic islet cell hyperplasia) Hypoglycemia, headache, weakness, perspiration, tachycardia, sweating, hunger, nervousness etc.
* **Hoffman's syndrome:**
  — *Hypothyroidism* ...muscular hypertrophy, weakness and slow ness of muscle contractions with normal EMG.
* **Kimmelsteil-Wilson Syndrome**
  — Diabetic glomerulosclerosis seen in diabetic patients.
* **Laron Syndrome:**
  — Pituitary dwarfism syndrome due to lack of production of somatomedin in response to GH.
* **Launois Syndrome:**
  (pituitary gigantism syndrome)
* **Nelson Syndrome:**
  (post-adrenalectomy syndrome)
* **Pseudo hypoparathyroidism syndrome:**
  (Chronic renal tubular insufficiency syndrome)
* **Sheehan's syndrome:**
  — Post-partum pituitary necrosis syndrome.
* **Simmond's syndrome:**
  — *Anterior pituitary gland lesions (due to injury, haemorrhage, infarction or tumours)*...progressive wt. loss, weakness, hypotension, anorexia, low body temp., anemia, dry skin with brittle nails, amenorrhoea and hypogonadism.
* **Bartter Syndrome (AR):**
  — Severe hypokalemmia due to excessive urinary K excretion leading to tetany, increased plasma renin, hyperaldosteronism and metabolic alkalosis, polyuria, polydipsia with normotension. Kidney biopsy shows juxtaglomerular and renal medullary hyperplasia.

CLASSIFICATION OF CAUSE OF HYPERCALCEMIA

Parathyroid-related:

1. Primary hyperparathyroidism
   a. Solitary adenomas
   b. Multiple endocrine neoplasia
2. Lithium therapy
3. Familial hypocalciuric hypercalcemia

Malignancy-related:

1. Solid tumor with metastases (breast)
2. Solid tumor with humoral mediation of hypercalcemia (lung, kidney)
3. Hematologic malignancies (multiple myeloma, lymphoma, leukemia)

Vitamin D—related:

1. vitamin D intoxication
2. 1,25(OH2)D; sarcoidosis and other granulomatous diseases
3. Idiopathic hypercalcemia of infancy

Associated with high bone turn over:

1. Hyperthyroidism
2. Immobilization
3. Thiazides
4. Vitamin A intoxication

Associated with renal failure:

1. Severe secondary hyperparathyroidism
2. Aluminium intoxication
3. Milk-alkali syndrome

HYPOTHALAMIC REGULATORY MECHANISMS.

Function	*Afferents From*	*Integrating Areas*
Temperature regulation	Cutaneous cold receptors; temperature-	Anterior hypothalamus, sensitive cells in hypothalamus
response to heat; posterior		hypothalamus, response to cold
Neuroendocrine control of: Catecholamines	Emotional stimuli, probably via limbic system	Dorsomedial and posterior hypothalamus
Vasopressin others	Osmoreceptors, "volume receptors",	Supraoptic and paraventricular nuclei
Oxytocin	Touch receptors in breast, uterus, genitalia	Supraoptic and paraventricular nuclei
Thyroid-stimulating hormone	Temperature receptors, perhaps others (?)	Anterior median eminence (TSH) and anterior hypothalamus
Adrenocorticotropic hormone (ACTH)	Limbic system (emotional stimuli); reticular formation ("systemic" stimuli); hypothalamic or anterior pituitary cells sensitive to circulating blood cortisol level; others (?)	Ventral hypothalamus
Follicle-stimulating hormone hormone (LH) Prolactin	Hypothalamic cells sensitive to estrogens; eyes, touch receptors in skin and genitalia of reflex ovulating species	Anterior hypothalamus, (FSH) and luteinizing other areas
	Touch receptors in breasts, other unknown receptors	Arcuate nucleus, median eminence (hypothalamus inhibits secretion)
Growth hormone	Unknown receptors	Anterior median eminence
"Appetitive" behavio		
Thirst	Osmoreceptors	Lateral superior hypothalamus

Hunger	"Glucostat" cells sensitive to rate of glucose utilization also limbic components	Ventromedial satiety center, lateral hunger center.
Sexual behavior	Cells sensitive to circulating estrogen and androgen, others cortex	Anterior ventral hypothalamus, plus, in the male, piriform
Defensive reactions Fear, rage	Sense organs and neocortex, paths unknown	Diffuse, in limbic system and hypothalamus
Control of various endocrine and activity rhythms	Retina via retinohypothalamic fibers	Suprachiasmatic nuclei

KNOWN AND SUSPECTED SYNAPTIC TRANSMITTER AGENTS AND "NEURAL HORMONES" IN MAMMALS.

Substance	*Known*	*Locations Where Substance Is Secreted Suspected*
Acetycholine	Myoneural junction Preganglionic autonomic endings Postganglionic parasympathetic endings Postganglionic sweat gland and muscle vasodilator endings Many parts of brain	Retina
Norepinephrine	Postganglionic sympathetic endings Cereral cortex, hypothalamus, brain stem, cerebellum, spinal cord	
Dopamine	Caudate nucleus, putamen, hypothalamus, limbic system, cerebral cortex	Retina
Epinephrine	Hypothalamus	
Serotonin	Hypothalamus, limbic system, cerebellum, spinal cord	Retina
Substance P	Substantia gelatinosa, many other parts of brain	Retina, intestine
Histamine		Hypothalamus
Vasopressin	Posterior pituitary	
Oxytocin	Posterior pituitary	
Hypothalamic releasing hormonem (CRH, TRH, GRH, GIH, LRH, FRH, PRH, PIH)	Median eminence of hypothalamus	Others parts of and inhibiting brain, spinal cord
Glycine		Neurons mediating direct inhibition in spinal cord
Gamma-aminobutyric acid(GABA)	Cerebral cortex; neurons mediating presynaptic inhibition in spinal cord; retina	

Glutamic acid (glutamate)	Excites many mammalian neurons
Enkephalins, endorphins	Many parts of CNS, gastrointestinal tract

THYROXINE-BINDING CAPACITY AND AFFINITY OF PLASMA PROTEIN CONSTITUENTS.

Protein	*Plasma Level (mg/dl)*	*Thyroxine-Binding Capacity (μg/dl)*	*Affinity for Thyroxine*	*Approximate Amount of Thyroxine Bound in Normal Plasma (μg/dl)*
Thyroxine-binding globulin (TBG)	1.0	20	High	7
Thyroxine-binding prealbumin (TBPA)	30.0	250	Moderate	1
Albumin	...	1000	Low	None
Total protein-bound thyroxine in plasma	...	...	...	8

EFFECT OF VARIATIONS IN THE CONCENTRATIONS OF THYROID HORMONE-BINDING PROTEINS IN THE PLASMA ON VARIOUS PARAMETERS OF THYROID FUNCTION.

	Concentrations of Binding Proteins	*Total Plasma T3 and T4*	*Free Plasma T3 and T4*	*Clinical State*
Hyperthyroidism	Normal	High	High	Hyperthyroid
Hypothyroidism	Normal	Low	Low	
Hypothyroid				
Pregnancy, estrogen treatment, congenital elevation of TBG	High	High	Normal	Euthyroid
Nephrosis, methyltestosterone, phenytoin, congenital depression of TBG	Low	Low	Normal	Euthyroid

SUMMARY OF CHEMICAL, ANATOMICAL AND PHARMACOLOGICAL CHARACTERISTICS OF THREE FAMILIES OF OPIOID PEPTIDES

Precursor	*Active peptide*	*Size (A.A.)*	*Distribution*	*Receptor Affinity*
Pro-opio melanocortin (POMC)	b-endorphin	31	Diffuse protection systems hypothalamus to limbic and brain stem areas	μ δ k
Proenkephalin	met-, leu-enkephalin	5	short interneurons; widely scattered including limbic system	δ
Pro-dynorphin	Dynorphines 1-17,1-8,1-9	17,8,9	Hypothalamus post. pitutary, basal ganglia, spinal cord	k

Relative potencies of corticosteroids. Values are approximations based on liver glucagon depletion or anti-inflammatory assays for glucocorticoid activity, and effect on urinary Na+/K+ or maintenance of adrenalectomized animals for mineralocorticoid activity. The last 3 steroids listed are synthetic compounds that do not occur naturally.

	Glucocorticoid Activity	*Mineralocorticoid Activity*
Cortisol	1.0	1.0
Corticosterone	0.3	15
Aldosterone	0.3	3000
Deoxycorticosterone	0.2	100
Cortisone	0.7	1.0
Prednisolone	4	0.8
9a-Fluorocortisol	10	125
Dexamethasone	25	~0

STIMULI WHICH INCREASE ALDOSTERONE SECRETION.

Glucocorticoid secretion also increased

- Surgery
- Anxiety
- Physical trauma
- Hemorrhage

Glucocorticoid secretion unaffected

- High potassium intake
- Low sodium intake
- Constriction of inferior vena cava in thorax
- Standing
- Secondary hyperaldosteronism (in some cases of congestive heart failure, cirrhosis, and nephrosis)

STIMULI THAT AFFECT GROWTH HORMONE SECRETION IN HUMANS.

Stimuli that increase secretion

Deficiency of energy substrate
- Hypoglycemia
- 2-Deoxyglucose
- Exercise
- Fasting

Increase in circulating levels of certain amino acids
- Protein meal
- Infusion of arginine and some other amino acids
- Glucagon
- Stressful stimuli
- Pyrogen
- Lysine vasopressin
- Various psychologic stresses
- Going to sleep
- L-Dopa
- Apomorphine

Stimuli that decrease secretion
- REM sleep
- Glucose
- Cortisol
- Free fatty acids
- Medroxyprogesterone
- Growth hormone

STIMULI THAT AFFECT GASTRIN SECRETION.

Stimuli that increase gastrin secretion

Luminal
- Peptides and amino acids
- Distention

Neural
- Increased vagal (cholinergic) discharge

Blood-borne
- Calcium
- Epinephrine

Stimuli that inhibit gastrin secretion

Luminal
- Acid

Blood-borne
- Secretin, GIP, VIP, glucagon, calcitonin

CLASSIFICATION OF TUMOR HYPERCALCEMIA

I. Hematologic malignancies
   a. Local bone destruction (QAF, interleukin 1, tumor necrosis factor, lymphotoxin)
      Multiple myeloma
      Lymphomas
   b. Humoral mediation [1,25(OH)2d, ?PTH-rP]
      Lymphomass
2. Solid tumors
   a. Local bone destruction (prostaglandin, E series)
      Breast carcinoma
   b. Humoral mediation (PTH-rP, ?other agents)
      Lung (squamous cell)
      Kidney
      Urogenital tract
      Other squamous tumors

FACTORS AFFECTING INSULIN SECRETION.

Stimulators	*Inhibitors*
Glucose	2-Deoxyglucose
Mannose	Mannoheptulose
Amino acids (leucine, arginine, others)	a-Adrenergic stimulating agents (norepinephrine, epinephrine)
b-Adrenergic blocking agents	b-Adrenergic stimulating agents (propranolol)
Acetylcholine	Diazoxide
Glucagon	Thiazide diuretics
Cyclic AMP and various cyclic AMP-generating substances	Phenytoin
Theophylline	Alloxan
Sulfonylureas	Microtubule inhibitors
Intestinal hormones (GIP, gastrin, secretin, CCK, glucagon, others?)	Somatostatin

FACTORS AFFECTING GLUCAGON SECRETION

Stimulators	*Inhibitors*
Amino acids (particularly the glucogenic amino acids : alanine, serine, glycine, cysteine and threonine)	Glucose
	Secretin
	FFA
	Ketones
CCK, gastrin	Phenytoin
b-Adrenergic Stimulation	a-Adrenergic stimulators
Theophylline	Somatostatin
Cortisol	
Exercise	
Infections	
Other stresses	

SUMMARY OF STIMULI AFFECTING VASOPRESSIN SECRETION.

Vasopressin Secretion Increased	*Vasopressin Secretion Decreased*
Increased effective osmotic pressure of plasma	Decreased effective osmotic ressure of plasma
Decreased extracellular fluid volume	Increased extracellular fluid volume
Morphine, nicotine, barbiturates	Alcohol
Pain, emotion, "stress", exercise.	

SOME HORMONES AND NEUROTRANSMITTERS THAT APPEAR TO EXERT THEIR EFFECTS BY INCREASING INTRACELLULAR CYCLIC AMP.

Catecholamines	Activation of phosphorylase in liver, heart, and skeletal muscle Lipolysis Positive inotropic response in heart Increased renin secretion Inhibition of Purkinje cell discharge in cerebellum
Glucagon	Activation of phosphorylase in liver Lipolysis Positive inotropic effect Stimulation of insulin secretion
Vasopressin	Increased water permeability of renal collecting duct epithelium
ACTH	Steroidogenesis in adrenal cortex
LH	Steroidogenesis in ovary and testis
TSH	Increased secretion of thyroid hormones
TRH and some other hypothalamic hormones	Increased secretion of anterior pituitary hormones
Parathyroid hormone	Increased Ca^{++} mobilization from bone Increased renal tubular reabsorption of Ca^{++}; increased PO_4^- excretion Increased intestinal absorption of Ca^{++}
Gastrin	Increased gastric secretion of hydrochloric acid
FSH	Actions on seminiferous tubules

EFFECT OF INSULIN ON GLUCOSE UPTAKE IN TISSUES IN WHICH IT HAS BEEN INVESTIGATED.

Tissues in which insulin facilitates glucose uptake

Skeletal muscle
Cardiac muscle
Smooth muscle
Adipose tissue
Leukocytes
Crystalline lens of the eye
Pituitary
Fibroblasts
Mammary gland
Aorta
A cells of pancreatic islets

Tissues in which insulin does not facilitate glucose uptake

Brain (except probably part of hypothalamus)
Kidney tubules
Intestinal mucosa
Red blood cells

PRINCIPAL ACTIONS OF INSULIN.

Adipose tissue

1. Increased glucose entry
2. Increased fatty acid synthesis
3. Increased glycerol phosphate synthesis
4. Increased triglyceride deposition
5. Activation of lipoprotein lipase
6. Inhibition of hormone-sensitive lipase
7. Increased potassium uptake

Muscle

1. Increased glucose entry
2. Increased glycogen synthesis
3. Increased amino acid uptake
4. Increased protein synthesis in ribosomes
5. Decreased protein catabolism
6. Decreased release of gluconeogenic amino acids
7. Increased ketone uptake
8. Increased potassium uptake

Liver

1. Decreased cyclic AMP
2. Decreased ketogenesis
3. Increased protein synthesis
4. Increased lipid synthesis
5. Decreased glucose output due to decreased gluconegenesis and increased glycogen synthesis

INSULIN/GLUCAGON MOLAR RATIOS (I/G) IN BLOOD IN VARIOUS CONDITIONS. 1+ TO 4 + INDICATE RELATIVE MAGNITUDE.

Condition	*Hepatic Glucose Storage (S) or Production (P)*	*I/G*
Glucose availability		
Large carbohydrate meal	4+(S)	70
IV glucose	2+(S)	25
Small meal	1+(S)	7
Glucose need		
Overnight need	1+(P)	2.3
Low carbohydrate diet	2+(P)	1.8
Starvation	4+(P)	0.4

TYPICAL PLASMA ELECTROLYTE LEVELS IN NORMAL HUMANS AND PATIENTS WITH ADRENOCORTICAL DISEASES.

	Plasma Electrolytes (mEq/liter)			
	Na^+	K^+	Cl^-	HCO_3^-
Normal	142	4.5	105	25
Adrenal insufficiency	120	6.7	85	25
Primary hyper-aldosteronism	148	2.4	96	41

STIMULI WHICH INCREASE ALDOSTERONE SECRETION.

Glucocorticoid secretion also increased

- Surgery
- Anxiety
- Physical trauma
- Hemorrhage

Glucocorticoid secretion unaffected

- High potassium intake
- Low sodium intake
- Constriction of inferior vena cava in thorax
- Standing
- Secondary hyperaldosteronism (in some cases of congestive heart failure, cirrhosis, and nephrosis)

DISTRIBUTION (MMOL/LITER) OF CALCIUM IN NORMAL HUMAN PLASMA.

Diffusible		1.34
Ionized (Ca^{++})	1.18	
Complexed to HCO_3^-, citrate, etc	0.16	
Nondiffusible (protein-bound)		1.16
Bound to albumin	0.92	
Bound to globulin	0.24	
Total plasma calcium		2.50

STIMULI WHICH INCREASE RENIN SECRETION.

- Sodium depletion
- Diuretics
- Hypotension
- Hemorrhage
- Upright posture
- Dehydration
- Constriction of renal artery or aorta
- Cardiac failure
- Cirrhosis

THE RENIN-ANGIOTENSIN-VASOCONSTRICTOR MECHANISM FOR ARTERIAL PRESSURE CONTROL.

1. Occurs rapidly—vasoconstriction especially of the arterioles and to a lesser extent of the veins at the same time. Constriction of the arterioles increases the peripheral resistance and thereby raises the arterial pressure back toward normal, as illustrated at the bottom of the schema.

2. Also, constriction of the veins increases the circulatory filling pressure, some times as much as 50 per cent, and this promotes increased tendency for venous return of blood to the heart to pump against the extra pressure load.

3. The other effects of angiotensin are mainly related to the body fluid volumes: (1) angiotensin has a direct effect on the kidneys to cause decreased excretion of both salt and water; and

   (2) angiotensin. stimulates the secretion of aldosterone by the adrenal cortex, and this hormone in turn also acts on the kidneys to cause decreased excretion of both salt and water. Both these effects elevate the blood volume—an important factor in long-term regulation of arterial pressure.

RELATIVE POTENCIES OF ADRENAL STEROIDS

		Approximate Relative Potency		
	Compound (tablet strength)	*Anti-inflammatory (Glucocorticoid) Effect*	*Sodium retaining (Mineralocorticoid) Effect*	*Equivalent Dosage (for Anti-inflammatory Effect)*
Cortisone	25 mg	0.8	1	25 mg
Hydrocortisone	20 mg	1.0	1	20 mg
Prednisolone and prednisone	5mg	4	0.8	5mg
Methyl-Prednisolone	4 mg	5	minimal	4 mg
Triamicinolone	4 mg	5	none	4 mg
Dexamethasone	0.5 mg	30	minimal	0.75 mg
Betamethasone	0.5 mg	30	negligible	0.7 mg
Paramethasone	2 mg	10	negligible	2 mg
Deoxycortone	—	negligible	50	—
Fludrocortisone	0.1 mg	15	150	—
Aldosterone	—	none	500	—

EQUIVALENT DOSES OF CORTICOSTEROIDS

Drug	*Dose*
Cortisone	25 mg
Hydrocortisone	20 mg
Prednisone and prednisolone	5 mg
Methylyprednisolone	4 mg
Dexamethasone	0.75 mg
Betamethasone	0.70 mg

GLUCOCORTICOID CORTICOSTEROIDS

	Equivalent dosage (mg)	*Mean dose to suppress HPA (mg/day)*	*Half-life in plasma (h)*	*Half-life of pharmacological effect (h)*
Hydrocortisone	20	15-30	1.5	8-12
Cortisone	25	20-35	1.5	8-12
Prednosolone	5	7.5-10	3+	18-36
Prednisone	5	7.5-10	3+	18-36
Methylprednisolone	4	7.5-10	3+	18-36
Dexamethasone	0.75	1-1.5	5+	36-54
Triamcinolone	4	7.5-10	3+	18-36
Betamethasone	0.6	1-1.5	5+	36-54

Progestins can also be classified on the basis of their biological characteristics :

I. *Pure progestins* e.g. Progesterone, Dehydrogesterone, Esters of 17-alpha hydroxyprogesterone, Chlormadinone and Megestrol.

II. *True progestins with possible androgenic effects* e.g. Medroxyprogesterone, Norgestrel,

III. *Progestins with androgenic effects* e.g. Norethisterone.

IV. *Progestins with estrogenic effects* e.g. Norethynodrol.

V. *Steroids of uncertain status* e.g. Ethynodiol diacetate.

*. DRUG INDUCED ENDOCRINE MANIFESTATIONS

A. Addisonian-like syndrome

Busulfan

Ketoconazole

B. Galactorrhea

Methyldopa
Phenothiazines
Reserpine
Tricyclic antidepressants

C. Gynecomastia

Calcium channel antagonists
Digitalis
Estrogens
Ethionamide
Griseofulvin
Isoniazid
Methyldopa
Phenytoin
Reserpine
Spironolactone
Testosterone

D. Thyroid function tests, disorders of

Acetazolamide
Amiodarone
Bomsulfophthalcin
Chlorpropamide
Clofibrate
Colestipol and nicotinic acid
Dimeraprol
Gold salts
Iodides
Lithium
Oral contraceptives
Phenindione
Phenothiazines (long-term)
Phenylbutazone
Phenytoin
Sulfomnamides
Tolbutamide

F. Vaginal carcinoma

Diethy Istilbestrol (given to mother)

APUD CELLS, APUDOMAS, AND ECTOPI POLYPEPTIDE HORMONES PRODUCED BY APUDOMAS

Cell	*Tumor*	*Putative Hormone*
Hypothalamic neurosecretory	Non identified	
Pinealocyte	Pinealoma	Unknown
Adenohypophyseal	Pituitary adenoma	Unknown
Autonomic neuron	Neurocytoma	ACTH; vasoactive intestinal peptide (VIP)
Chromaffin	Pheochromocytoma	ACTH; follicle-stimulating hormone; calcitonin (CT); insulin
Carotid-body and other paraganglion cells	Paraganglioma; chemodectoma	ACTH; CT
Thyroid C	Meduallary carcinoma of thyroid	ACTH; insulin
Bronchial Kulchitsky	Bronchial carcinoid; oat cell carcinoma	ACTH; ADH; CT glucagon; insulin; growth hormone; prolactin
Gastrointestinal endocrine	Intestinal carcinoid	ACTH; ADH
Pancreatic islet	Islet cell tumor	ACTH; ADH; VIP
Melanocyte	Melanoma	ACTH; gastrin

SPECTRUM OF ECTOPIC HORMONE PRODUCTION

Tumor Type Group/hormone	*Common*	*Infrequent*
1. Neuroendocrine-gastrointestinal		
a. ACTH, β lipotropin, endorphins, MSHs, enkephalins	Lung carcinoma (small cell) Thymoma Pancreatic islet tumors Carcinoid Thyroid medullary carcinoma Pheochromocytoma Parotid tumor Prostatic carcinoma Renal carcinoma	Squamous cell, adenocarcinoma, and large cell carci noma of the lung Breast carcinoma Colonic carcinoma Gallbladder tumors Testicular carcinoma Uterine carcinoma Laryngeal carcinoma Plasmacytoma Bladder small cell carcinoma
b. Vasopressin, oxytocin, neurophysin	Lung carcinoma (small cell, anaplastic adenocarcinoma)	Pancreatic carcinoma Duodenal carcinoma

Tumor Type Group/hormone	*Common*	*Infrequent*
c. Corticotropin-releasing hormone	Lung carcinoma (small cell) Carcinoid	Pituitary gangliocytoma Medullary carcinoma of thyroid
d. Growth hormone releasing hormone	Carcinoid Pancreatic islet adenoma Lung carcinoma (small cell)	Adrenocortical adenoma Neurofibroma Endometrial carcinoma Pheochromocytoma Pituitary gangliocytoma
e. Somatostatin	Lung carcinoma (small cell) Carcinoid	
f. Calcitonin	Lung carcinoma (small cell) Carcinoid	Breast carcinoma Pheochromocytoma
g. Gastrin	Lung carcinoma (small cell)	Ovarian carcinoma
h. Vasoactive intestinal peptide	Lung carcinoma (small cell) Pancreatic islet tumors	
i. Insulin	Lung carcinoma Carcinoid	Gastric carcinoma
j. Glucagon		Lung carcinoma Carcinoid Renal carcinoma
k. Gastrin-releasing peptide (bombesin-like)	Lung carcinoma Carcinoid	Medullary carcinoma of thyroid
2. Fetoplacental and/or anterior pituitary		
a. Chorionic gonadotropin (and subunits)	Lung carcinoma Gastric carcinoma *Ovarian carcinoma Adeno-and islet cell carcinoma of the pancreas Hepatoma	Testicular carcinoma Ovarian carcinoma Adenocortical carcinoma Breast carcinoma Melanoma Carcinoid
b. Placental lactogen Hepatoma	Lung carcinoma (small cell)	Lymphoma Pheochromocytoma
c. Growth hormone		Lung carcinoma (large cell) Carcinoid Pancreatic islet tumor
d. Prolactin		Lung carcinoma Renal carcinoma Gonadoblastoma
3. Others		
a. Tissue growth factors (somatomedins)	Mesenchymal tumors (i.e., fibrosarcoma) Hepatoma Adenocortical carcinoma Pancreatic/bile duct carcinoma	Lung carcinoma Ovarian carcinoma Neuroblastoma Wilms's tumor

SPECTRUM OF ECTOPIC HORMONE PRODUCTION (Contd..)

Tumor Type Group/hormone	Common	Infrequent
b. Erythropoietin	Cerebellar hemangioblastoma Uterine fibroma Renal carcinoma	Adenocortical carcinoma. Hepatoma Pheochromocytoma
c. Humoral hypercalcemic factor of malignancy, osteoclast-activating factor	Renal carcinoma Lung carcinoma (squamous) Hepatoma Pancreatic islet tumors	GI tract tumors Parotid tumors Genitourinary tumors Melanoma Breast carcinoma
d. 1, 25 Dihydroxy vitamin D	Lymphoma	

PHYSIOLOGIC ABNORMALITIES DUE TO NEOPLASIA—ENDOCRINE SYNDROMES DUE TO ECTOPIC HORMONE SECRETION

Clinical Manifestations	*Neoplasm*
HYPERADRENAL CORTICISM due to ectopic ACTH secretion or "corticortrophin-releasing	Small cell cancer of lung, thymoma, carcinoid tumors, cancers of breast, ovary, factor" secretion prostate
HYPERTHYROIDISM due to ectopic TSH secretion, Manifestations generally mild	Choriocarcinoma, placental tumors, embryonal cancer of testis.
HYPOGLYCEMIA due to ectopic secretion of insulin like hormone, impaired glycogenolysis, excessive glucose consumption by tumor, under alimentation or combined factors	Retroperitoneal and intrathroacic tumors, Sarcoma, lymphoma, melanoma
HYPOGLYCEMIA due to excessive secretion of HGH, catecholamines, glucagon, adrenal steroids, estrogens; body wasting	Several tumor types
FEMINZATION—SEXUAL PRECOCITY—due to ectopic gonadotrophin secretion	Bronchogenic cancer, esp. giant cell. Teratomas, breast cancer, melanoma
VIRILIZATION—SEXUAL PRECOCITY due to ectopic gonadotrophin or ACTH secretion	Several tumor types, hepatoblastoma, melanoma, cancers of breast and lung.

PANCREATIC ENDOCRINE TUMORS

Syndrome	*Hormone(s) produced*	*Primary hormone effects*	*Pathologic features*	*Clinical features*
Zollinger-Ellison	Gastrin	Gastric acid hypersecretion with basal acid outputs usually > 15 mmol/h (>15 meq/h)	Delta cell islet tumors, 10% aberrrant (duodenal); 60% malignant	Severe peptic ulcer disease often refractory to therapy, ectopic ulcers, diarrhea; multiple endocrine adenomas (parathyroid, pituitary, adre- thyroid)
nal, Insulinoma	Insulin	Hypoglycemia with inappropriately increased serum insulin levels	Beta cell islet tumors; 80-90% benign	Hypoglycemic symptoms
Glucagonoma	Glucagon; pancreatic poly-peptide	Hyperglucagonemia, glucose intolerance	Alpha cell islet tumors, 60% malignant	Slow-growing pancreatic tumor; hyperglycemia, bullous and eczematoid dermatitis, weight loss, anemia; gastric and intestinal motor abnormalities
Somatostatinoma	Somatostatin; pancreatic polypeptide	Somatostatin inhibits insulin, gastrin and pancreatic and bile flow	Delta cell islet tumor	Pancreatic tumor; diarrhea; steatorrhea; gallstones; diabetes mellitus; anemia.
Pancreatic cholera	Vasoactive intestinal peptide(VIP) ?Gastric inhibtory polypeptide ?Prostaglandin E ?Pancreatic peptide	Net secretion of salt and water by gut	? Delta cell tu* > 50% malignant	Pancreatic tumor with severe watery diarrhea; flushing; weight loss; hypokalemia; hypercalcemia; hypochlorhydria; hyperglycemia; inordinate fecal water and electrolyte losses
Carcinoid	Serotonin; prostaglandin	Altered gut motility; diarrhea	Enteochromaffin cells; non-beta cell islet tumors	Carcinoid syndrome with flushing; wheezing; diarrhea; alcohol intolerance; hepatomegaly

DISTRIBUTION OF APUD TUMORS

Origin	*Tumors*
Gastrointestinal tract	Carcinoid tumor
Pancreas	Islet cell carcinoma
Central nervous system	Ganglioneuroblastoma, neuroblastoma, chemodactoma, paraganglionoma
Thyroid	Medullary thyroid carcinoma
Skin	Melanoma
Adrenal medulla	Pheochromocytoma
Lung	Carcinoid tumor, small cell carcinoma

GASTROINTESTINAL ENDOCRINE TUMOR SYNDROMES

Syndrome	*Cell type*	*Clinical features*	*Percentage malignant*	*Major products*
Carcinoid syndrome	Enterochromaffin, entero-chromaffin-like	Flushing, diarrhea, wheezing, hypotension	*100	Serotonin, hitamine, miscellaneous peptides
Zollinger-Ellison, gastrinoma	Non-β islet cell, duodenal G cell	Peptic ulcers, diarrhea	*70	Gastrin
Insulinoma	Islet βcell	Hypoglycemia	* 10	Insulin
Verner-Morrison, WDHa, VIPoma, pancreatic cholera	Islet β cell	Diarrhea, hypokalemia, hypochlorhydria	*60	Vasoactive intestintal peptide
Glucagonoma	Islet A cell	Mild diabetes mellitus, erythema necrolytics migrans, glossitis	>75	Glucagon
Somatostatinoma	Islet D cell	Diabetes mellitus, diarrhea, steatorrhea, gallstones	-70	Somatostatin
GRFoma	Non β ilset cell	Acromegaly	—	Growth hormone-releasing hormone (GRF)
CRFoma	Non-β- islet cell	Cushing's syndrome	—	Corticotropin-releasing hormone (CRF)
PPoma	Islet PP cell	Rare necrolytic erythema	—	Pancreatic polypeptide (PP)
Neurotensinoma	Non-β islet cell	None	—	Neurotensin
Miscellaneous tumors	Non-β islet cell	Hypercalcemia	—	Parathyroid hormone
		Inappropriate ADH	—	Vasopressin
		Hyperpigmentation	—	Melanocyte-stimulating hormone

CLUES TO THE PRESENCE OF ENDOCRINE DYSFUNCTION

Sign or Symptom	*Metabolic Disorder*
Skin	
Excess hair growth	Adrenal hyperplasia or tumor Stein-Leventhal syndrome Ovarian tumor Obesity Adrenal hypersensitivity
Pruritus	Diabetes mellitus, hyperthyroidism, uremia
Vitiligo hypo-and	Adrenal insufficiency, Hashimoto's thyroiditis, diabetes, hyperthyrodism
Excess sweat	Hyperthyroidism, pheochromocytoma, acromegaly,
Hypoglycemia	
Flushing	Pheochromocytoma and carcinoid syndrome
Increased pigment	Addison's disease, hyperthyroidism
Cold skin	Myxedema, pheochromocytoma
Ecchymoses	Cushing's syndrome
Central Nervous System	
Headache	Pituitary tumors, hypoglycemia, pheochromocytoma
Psychosis	Hypoglycemia, thyrotoxicosis, myxedema, Cushing's syndrome, hyponatremia, hyperparathyroidism

Fatigue	Adrenal insufficiency, hypoglycemia, acromegaly, hyper- and hypothyroidism
Ataxia	Myxedema
Somnolence, coma	Diabetic acidosis, hypercalcemia, myxedema, hypoglycemia, hyperglycemia, hyponatremia
Paresthesias	Myxedema, hypocalcemia, acromegaly, diabetes mellitus
Ear, Nose, Throat	
Deafness, tinnitus, nasal congestion, excess cerumen	Myxedema
Ocular	
Diplopia	Hyperthyroidism, diabetes mellitus
Bitermporal hemianopsia	Pituitary tumors (acromegaly, etc)
Cardiovascular	
Hypertension	Hyperaldosteronism, Cushing's syndrome, hypercalcemia, myxedema, acromegaly, pheochromocytoma
Tachycardia or atrial fibrillation	Thyrotoxicosis, pheochromocytoma
Congestive failure	Thyrotoxicosis, Cushing' syndrome
Venous thromboses	Hypercalcemia
Pericardial effusion	Myxedema
Bradycardia	Myxedema
Hypotension	Adrenal insufficiency
Gastrointestinal	
Dyspepsia	Hypercalcemia, myxedema, adrenal insufficiency
Peptic ulcer	Hyperparathyrodism, islet cell tumor
Diarrhea	Hyperthyroidism, diabetes mellitus. adrenal insufficency, hypocalcemia, islet cell tumor
Anorexia	Hypercalcemia, adrenal insufficieny, myxedema
Weight loss	Adrenal insufficiency, hyperthyroidism, pheochromocytoma
Constipation	Myxedema, hypercalcemia, pheochromocytoma
Ascites	Myxedema
Abdominal pain	Adrenal insufficiency, hyperlipemia, hyperparathyroidism
Urological	
Polyuria, polydipsia	Hypercalcemia, hyperaldosteronism, pituitary tumor, diabetes mellitus
Kidney stones	Hyperparathyroidism, Cushing's syndrome, acromegaly, gout, cystinuria
Musculoskeletal	
Weakness	Hyperthyroidism, Cushing's syndrome. acromegaly, hyperparathyroidism
Arthralgia	Myxedema, acromegaly

Bone pain	Hyperparathyroidism
Fractures	Cushing's syndrome hyperparathyroidism
Genital	
Menorrhagia	Hyperthyroidism
Metrorrhagia	Myxedema
Loss of libido and potenita	Hypogonadism, acromegaly, hypothyroidism, diabetes mellitus
Amenorrhea	Hyperthyroidism, hypogonadism, Cushing's syndrome, acromegaly, pituitary tumor, Sheehan's syndrome
Laboratory Findings	
Hyponatremia	Addison's disease, hypopituitarism, hypothyroidism, ADH excess
Anemia	Mxedema, adrenal insufficiency, hyperparathyroidism, hyperthyroidism
Hypokalemia	Hyperaldosteronism, ectopic ACTH syndrome, Cushing's syndrome
Hypocalcemia	Hypoparathyroidism, magnesium deficiency
Hypoglycemia	Islet cell tumor, functional hyperinsulinism, early diabetes mellitus, adrenal insufficiency, growth hormone deficiency
Hyperlipemia	Pancreatitis, lipidoses, Cushing's syndrome, myxedema

SOMATOSTATIN

Somatostatin inhibits release of:	*Sites of production:*
* GH	* Hypothalamus
* Gastrin	* Gastrointestinal tract
* TSH	* Delta cells of pancreas
* Glucagon	
* Gastric acid	
* Insulin	
* Pancreatic enzymes	

DIFFERENTIAL DIAGNOSIS OF SHORT STATURES

Impaired growth velocity

* *Endocrine*
  Isolated GH deficiency
  Panhypopituitarism
  Primary hypothyroidism
  Cushing's syndrome

* *Abnormal body proportions*
  Short limbs for spine (e.g. achondroplasia)
  Short limbs and very short spine (e.g. mucopolysac-charidoses)
* *Other conditions*
  Chromosome abnormalities (e.g. Turner's)
  Malabsorption (coeliac, Crohn's colitis)
  Systemic illness (asthma, heart, renal disease)
  Malnutrition
  Psychosocial deprivation

Normal growth velocity on presentation

* Prior problem affecting growth but no longer active
  Intra-uterine growth retardation
  Congenital heart disease
* Constitutional short stature
  Normal bone age
* Physiological growth delay
  Retarded bone age

ACROMEGALY—MANIFESTATIONS

Location	*Symptoms*	*Signs*
General	Fatigue Increased sweating Heat intolerance Weight gain	
Skin and subcutaneous tissue	Enlarging hands, feet Coarsening facial features Oily skin Hypertrichosis	Moist, warm, fleshy, doughy handshake Skin tags Acanthosis nigricans Increased heel pad
Head	Headaches	Parotid enlargement, frontal bossing
Eyes	Decreased vision	Visual field defects
Ears		Otoscope speculum cannot be inserted
Nose-throat-paranasal sinuses	Sinus congestion	Enlarged furrowed tongue
	Increased tongue size	Tooth marks on tongue
	Malocclusion	Widely spaced teeth
	Voice change	Prognathism
		Goiter

Neck		Obstructive sleep apnea Enlarged sinuses
Cardiorespiratory system	Congestive heart failue	Hypertension Cardiomegaly Left ventricular hypertrophy
Genitourinary system	Decreased libido Impotence Oligomenorrhea Infertility Kidney stones	
Neurologic system	Paresthesias Hypersomnolence	Carpal tunnel syndrome
Muscles	Weakness	Proximal myopathy
Skeletal system	Joint pains (shoulder, back, knees)	Osteoarthritis

CAUSES OF HYPOPITUITARISM

A. Isolated hormone deficiencies
   I. Congenital or acquired deficiencies

B. Tumors
   1. Large pituitary adenomas
   2. Pituitary apoplexy
   3. Hypothalamic tumors, e.g., craniopharyngiomas, germinomas, chordomas, meningiomas, gliomas, and others

C. Inflammatory diseases
   1. Granulomatous disease, e.g., sarcoidosis, tuberculosis, syphilis, granulomatous hypophysitis
   2. Eosinophilic granuloma
   3. Lymphocytic hypophysitis (autoimmune)

D. Vascular diseases
   1. Sheehan's postpartum necrosis
   2. ? Diabetic peripartum necrosis
   3. Carotid aneurysm

E. Destructive-traumatic events
   1. Surgery
   2. Stalk section
   3. Radiation (conventional—hypothalamus; heavy-particle—pituitary)
   4. Trauma

F. Developmental anomalies
   1. Pituitary aplasia
   2. Basal encephalocoele
G. Infiltration
   1. Hemochromatosis
   2. Amyloidosis
H. "Idiopathic" causes
   1. ? Autoimmune disease

CAUSES OF SIADH

1. Malignant neoplasms with autonomous AVP release
   A. Oat cell carcinoma of lung
   B. Carcinoma of pancreas
   C. Lymphosarcoma, reticulum cell sarcoma, Hodgkin's dis ease
   D. Carcinoma of duodenum
   E. Thymoma
II. Nonmalignant pulmonary diseases
   A. Tuberculosis
   B. Lung abscess
   C. Pneumonia
   D. Viral pneumonitis
   E. Empyema
   F. Chronic obstructive airways disease
III. Central nervous system disorders
   A. Skull fracture
   B. Subdural hematoma
   C. Subarachnoid hemorrhage
   D. Cerebral vascular thrombosis
   E. Cerebral atrophy
   F. Acute encephalitis
   G. Tuberculous meningitis
   H. Purulent meningitis
   I. Guillain-Barre syndrome
   J. Lupus erythematosus
   K. Acute intermittent porphyria
IV. Drugs
   A. Chlorpropamide

B. Vincristine
C. Vinblastine
D. Cyclophosphamide
E. Carbamazepine
F. Oxytocin
G. General anesthesia
H. Narcotics
I. Tricyclic antidepressants

V. Miscellaneous causes
A. Hypothyroidism
B. Positive pressure respiration

CAUSES OF NEPHROGENIC DIABETES INSIPIDUS

This may be due to:

* *Genetic defect*
Sex-linked recessive
Cystinosis

* *Metabolic abnormality*
Hypokalaemia
Hypercalcaemia

* *Drug therapy*
Lithium
Demethylchloretracycline

* *Poisoning*
Heavy metals

STATES ASSOCIATED WITH DECREASED PERIPHERAL CONVERSION OF T4 TO T3

I. Physiologic
A. Fetal and early neonatal life
B. ? Old age

II. Pathologic
A. Fasting
B. Malnutriton
C. Systemic illness
D. Physical trauma
E. Postoperative state
F. Drugs (prophylthiouracil, dexamethasone, propranolol, amiodarone)
G. Radiographic contrast agents (idopanoic acid)

FACTORS AFFECTING THYROID BINDING GLOBULIN

*TBG Increased **

Pregnancy	Hypothroidism
Estrogens	Early Acute Hepatitis
Oral Contraceptives	Cirrhosis
Newborn	Acute Intermittent Porphyria
Trilafon	Genetic TBG Excess

*TBG Decreased**

Androgens	Nephrotic Syndrome
Anabolic Steroids	Type III Hyperlipoproteinemia
Phenylbutazone	
Hyperthyroidism	Chronic Metabolic Acidosis
Active Acromegaly	Severe Acute or Chronic
Klinefelter's Syndrome	Nonthyroidal illness
Down's Syndrome	Major Surgery
	Cushing's Syndrome
	Genetic TBG Deficiency

Competitors With Thyroxine For TBG Binding

Triiodothyronine	Dicumarol
Dilantin*	Atromid-S*
Heparin	D-Thyroxine

* *Thyrometabolic evaluation should include a free T4 or FT4 if a disparity between the clinical and laboratory picture exists.*

CLINICAL FEATURES OF HYPERTHYROIDISM

Goitre

Diffuse ± bruit

Nodular

Gastrointestinal

Weight loss despite normal or increased appetite

Hyperdefaecation

Diarrhoea and steatorrhoea

Anorexia

Vomiting

Cardiorespiratory
Palpitations, sinus tachycardia, atrial fibrillation3
Increased pulse pressure
Ankle oedema in absence of cardiac failure
Angina, cardiomyopathy and cardiac failure
Dyspnoea on exertion
Exacerbation of asthma
Neuromuscular
Nervousness, irritability, emotional lability, psychosis
Tremor
Hyper-reflexia, ill-sustained clonus
Muscle weakness, proximal myopathy, bulbar myopathy
Periodic paralysis (predominantly Chinese)
Dermatological
Increased sweating, pruritus
Palmar erythema, spider naevi
Onycholysis
Alopecia
Pigmentation, vitilligo
Finger clubbing
Pretibial myxoedema
Reproductive
Amenorrhoea/oligomenorrhoea
Infertility, spontaneous abortion
Loss of libido, impotence
Ocular
Lid, retraction, lid lag
Grittiness, corneal ulceration
Chemosis
Papilloedema, loss of visual acuity
Other
Heat intolerance
Fatigue, apathy
Gyanecomastia
Lymphadenopathy

Thirst

1 Features of Graves disease only.
2 The most common symptoms of hyperthyroidism, irrespective of its cause.
3 Features found particularly in elderly patients.

DIFFERENTIATING THE TYPES OF HYPERTHYROIDISM

Type	*Criteria for Diagnosis*
Toxic Diffuse Goite	Ophthalmopathy, Dermopathy
	RAIU*: Elevated or Normal ** T4, elevated T3
	Suppression Test: Abnormal***
Toxic Nodular Goiter	Thyroid Scintiscan: Solitary hot nodule (uninodular), Multiple hot nodules (Type I multinodular), Nonhomogenuous (Type II multinodular)
	T3 Suppression Test: Abnormal
	TSH Stimulation Test: Demonstrating the normal suppressed thyroid gland in uninodular and Type I multinodular
Toxic Thyroid Carcinoma	Proven thyroid carcinoma, thyroid and body
	^{131}I Scan: Positive for active metastatic lesions
Toxic Struma Ovarii	Abrominal mass with or without ascites
	RAIU: Low, rarely normal
	PB131I: High
	Abdominal 131 I Scan: Positive
	Hyperthyroidism Associated With Thyroiditis Tender Thyroid and/or constitutional signs and symptoms (fever, malaise, etc)
Acute Nonsuppurative	RAIU:Low
	Thyroid Antibodies: Low or absent
Chronic Lymphocytic	Thyroid Antibodies: High Titers
Hyperthyroidism Induced By	Long-standing nontoxic multinodular goiter with or without iodine deficiency
Exogenous Iodine	RAIU: Low
	Plasma Inorganic Iodide: Elevated
Thyrotoxicosis Due To TSH or TSH-like Substance	
TSH Excess	Signs and symptoms of pituitary disease
	TSH-RIA: Elevated
TSH-Like Substance	Abdominal or testicular mass
	TSH-Bioassay: Elevated
	TSH-RIA: Normal or Low
	HCG: High titers (hydatidiform mole and choriocarcinoma)

Hyperthyroidism Due To Exogenous Thyroid Hormone	RAIU: Low PBI^{131}: Low

* Required only in absence of pathonomonic physical findings

** In T3 toxicosis

*** Required when other measures are equivocal

RAIU—radioactive iodine uptake PBI^{131}—protein bound iodine131. TSH-RIA—thyroid Stimulating Hormone by Radio-immunoassay, HCG— Human Chorionic Gonadotrophin.

CLINICAL FEATURES OF HYPOTHYROIDISM

General

Tiredness, somnolence
Weight gain
Cold intolerance
Hoarseness
Goitre

Cardiorespiratory

Bradycardia, hypertension, angina, cardiac failure*
Xanthelasma
Pericardial and pleural effusion*

Neuromuscular

Aches and pains, muscle stiffness
Delayed relaxation of tendon reflexes
Carpal tunnel syndrome, deafness
Depression, psychosis*
Cerebellar ataxia*
Myotonia*

Haematological

Macrocytosis
Anaemia
- Iron deficiency (pre-menopausal women)
- Normochromic
- Pernicious

Dermatological

Dry flaky skin and hair, alopecia

Purplish lips and malar flush, carotenaemia

Vitiligo

Erythema ab igne (Granny's tartan)

Myxoedema

Reproductive

Menorrhagia

Infertility

Galactorrhea*, impotence*

Gastrointestinal

Constipation

Ileus*

Ascites*

* Rare but well-recognised features.

DIFFERENTIATING THE TYPES OF HYPOTHYROIDISM

Type of Primary Hypothyroidism	*Criteria for Diagnosis*
Iodine Deficiency	Endemic or Sporadic
RAIU: Elevated	
Plasma Inorganic Iodine: Low	
Iodine Excess	Plasma Inorganic Iodine: Elevated
RAIU: Low	
Multinodular Colloid Goiter	Thyroid scan: nonhomogeneous uptake
Thyroid Antibodies: Absent	
Inherited Defects In Hormonogenesis	
Type I	RAIU: Absent Thyroid and Salivary Gland Scintiscan: No demonstrable tissue Saliva: Serum I^{131} Ration: <10
Type II	RAIU: 2 or 4 hr—elevated, 24 hr—less than 2 or 4 hr Perchlorate Discharge Test: abnormal
Type III	RAIU: Elevated Chromatograph of thyroid tissue: excess MIT and DIT decreased T4 and T3
Type IV	RAIU: Elevated Intravenous Radioiodine Labeled MIT and DIT: appears in urine unchanged

Type V	RAIU: Elevated Thyroid Biopsy: absent thyroglobulin with 3S to 8S subunits immunologically demonstrable
Chronic Lymphocytic Thyroiditis	Dysphagia, dyspnea, and/or dysphonia, thyroid gland rock hard Thyroid biopsy: diagnostic
Goitrogen Induced Hypothyroidism	Identification of goitrogen
Postablative Hypothyroidism	History of thyroid surgery and/or radioiodine therapy
Type of Secondary Hypothyroidism	
Pituitary Disease	TRH Stimulation Test: abnormal
Hypothalamic and/or Hypophyseal Portal System Disease	TRH Stimulation Test: normal

RAIU-radioactive iodine uptake, MIT-monoiodotyrosine-DIT-diiodotyrosine, TRH-Thyrotrophin releasing Hormone

THE HORMONES OF THE ADRENAL CORTEX

	Cortisol	*Aldosterone*	*Adrenal Androgen*
			D4-androstenedione Dehydroepiandrosterone (DHA) 11-hydroxy-D4-androstenedione
Zone of Origin	Zona fasciculata	Zona glomerulosa	Zona reticularis
Secretion Rate	15-30 g per day	50-200 mg per day	DHA: 15-25 mg per day
Plasma Concentration	AM 15-25 mg per 100 ml PM 5-10 mg per 100 ml	4-8 mg per 100 ml	DHA: 0.4-0.6 mg per 100 ml
Relative potency			D4-androstenedione = 100% 11-hydroxy-D4-androstenedione = 5% DHA = 25%
Degradation products	Tetrahydrocortisol, tetrahydrocortisone, allotetrahydrocortisol Cortol, cortolone 11-oxy 17-ketosteroids	Tetrahydroaldosterone Conjugated active aldosterone Other compounds	Androsterone (5a) Etiocholanolone (5ß) DHA, unchanged (3 ß)
Methods for Urinary Measurements			
Commonest	Porter-Silber reaction (colorimetric reaction with phenylhydrazine)	Immunoassay or double-isotope derivative assay	Zimmerman reaction (colorimetric, reaction with m-dinitrobenzene, in the presence of alcoholic KOH)
Measures	17,21-dihydroxy, 20-ketone	Aldosterone-18-glucuronide	17-keto group (keto group at C3 and C20 also contributes)
Normal	4-10 mg per day	1-15 mg per day	Males 10-15 mg per day Females 5-10 mg per day
Other methods	Urinary free cortisol, 17-ketogenic steroids	Soda-fluorescence	DHA, a 3 ß-OH compound is precipitated by digitonin Hence 3a-and 3ß-17KS can be distin guished
Stimulus for Secretion by Adrenal	ACTH	Changes in effective plasma volume and potassium concentration mediated via renin—angiotension system Others including ACTH	ACTH ? other pituitary trophic hormones (?LH)

Actions	*Metabolic* Hyperglycemic Protein Fat redistribution Potassium movement from muscle (?) *Renal* Maintenance of normal GFR; excretion of normal water load Enhances sodium reabsorption at distal tubule Potassium diuresis *Inflammation* Decreases permeability of vessels Makes connective tissues nonresponsive to hyaluronidase Lymphocytolysis Preservation of lysosome membrane	*Renal* Enhances Na+ reabsorption from ascending loop of Henle Enhances Na^+ reabsorption, by exchange with K^+ and H^+, in distal convoluted tubule Enhances Na^+ exchange for NH^+4 in collecting duct *Extrarenal* Decreases Na: K ratio in saliva and in sweat glands	Body hair: pubic and axillary Sebaceous glands: secretions more oily Anabolic: nitrogen retaining effects Contributes to skeletal maturation

FACTORS REGULATING ALDOSTERONE BIOSYNTHESIS

	Factors	*Effects*
I	Renin-angiotensin system	Stimulate
II	Sodium ion	Inhibit (?physiologic)
III	Potassium ion	Stimulate
IV	Neurotransmitters	
	A. Dopamine	Inhibit
	B. Serotonin	Stimulate
V	Pituitary hormones	
	A. ACTH	
	B. Non-ACTH pituitary hormones (e.g., growth hormone)	Permissive (for optimal response to sodium restriction)
	C. Unidentified pituitary factors	Stimulate
	D. Beta endorphin	Stimulate
	E. g-MSH	Permissive
VI	Natriuretic factors	
	A. Atrial peptide	Inhibit
	B. Ouabain-like factors	Inhibit

RANGE OF NORMAL VALUES FOR TEST OF ADRENAL FUNCTION

Test	*Normal value, range*
Plasma, cortisol, nmol/L (m/dL):	
8 A.M.	140-690 (5-24)
4 P.M.	80-330 (3-12)
Cortisol secretory rate, nmol/d (mg/d)	14-69 (5-25)
Urinary free cortisol, nmol/d (mg/d)	55-275 (20-100)
17-Hydroxycorticosteroids, mmol/d (mg/d)	5.5-28 (2-10)
Plasma testosterone, nmol/L (ng/mL):	
Men	10-35 (3-10)
Women	<3.5 (<1)
Plasma dehydroepiandrosterone (DHEA) nmol/L (μg/L)	7-31 (2-9)
Plasma DHEA sulfate, mmol/L (mg/L)	1.3-6.7 (500-2500)
Plasma 11-deoxycortisol (S), nmol/L (mg/dL)	<30 (<1)
Plasma 17 OH progesterone, nmol/L (mg/L):	
Women	
Follicular phase	0.6-3 (0.2-1)
Luteal phase	1.5-10.6 (0.5-3.5)
Men	0.2-9 (0.06-3)
Plasma aldosterone, pmol/L (ng/dL) (100 mmol Na, 60-100 mmol K, supine, 8 A.M.)	< 240 (<8)
Aldosterone secretion nmol/d (mg/d) (100 Na, 600-100 mmol K)	140-690 (50-250)
Aldosterone excretion, nmol/d (mg/d) (100 mmol Na, 60-100 mmol K)	14-53 (5-19)
Plasma renin activity (mg/d)/h [(ng/mL)/h] (100 mmol Na, 60-100 mmol K, supine, 8 A.M.	1-2.5 (1-2.5)
Plasma angiotensin II ng/L (pg/mL) (100 mmol Na, 60-100 mmol K, supine, 8 A.M.)	10-30 (10-30)
Plasma ACTH, pmol/L (pg/mL) (8 A.M.)	<18 (<80)

CAUSES OF CUSHING'S SYNDROME

I. Adrenal hyperplasia
   A. Secondary to pituitary ACTH overproduction
      1. Pituitary-hypothalamic dysfunction
      2. Pituitary ACTH-producing micro- or macroadenomas

B. Secondary to ACTH or CRH-producing nonendocrine tumors (bronchogenic carcinoma, carcinoid of the thymus, pancreatic carcinoma, bronchial adenoma)

II. Adrenal nodular hyperplasia

III. Adrenal neoplasia

A. Adenoma

B. Carcinoma

IV. Exogenous, iatrogenic causes

A. Prolonged use of glucocorticoids

B. Prolonged use of ACTH

CLINICAL-METABOLIC CORRELATES IN CUSHING'S SYNDROME

I. Metabolic Effects

A. Fat Metabolism

Truncal obesity, widening of mediastinum

Hypercholesterolemia, accelerated atherosclerosis

B. Protein Metabolism

Muscle wasting with proximal myopathy

Fragility of skin—ecchymoses, striae

Growth hormone unresponsiveness

C. Carbohydrate Metabolism

Latent or overt diabetes mellitus

D. Electrolyte Balance

Aldosterone or DOC excesss with hypertension, hypokalemic alkalosis

II. Endocrine Effects

A. 1.25 Dihydroxycholecalciferol antagonism—secondary PTH excess and osteopenia

B. Growth Hormone suppression—growth failure

C. MSH Excess—hyperpigmentation

D. Androgen excess—hirsutism, amenorrhea, and infertility.

III. Neurologic

A. Psychosis or emotional lability

DIAGNOSIS OF CUSHING'S SYNDROME

Critical Questions	*Specific Tests*	*Comment*
Is hypercorticism possible?	Cushingoid habitus Hypertension Diabetes mellitus	Not selective criteria
Is hypercorticism likely?	Ecchymoses Muscle weakness Hypokalemia Osteoporosis	Obesity of arms or legs is against the diagnosis
Laboratory confirmation	Abnormal low dose or overnight dexamethasone suppression tests	Suppression urinary 17-OHCS above 2 mg per24 hours, urinary free cortisol above 20 mg per 24 hours 8 A.M. plasma corticoids above 10 mg/100 ml
above		High urinary free corticoids Control urinary free cortisol 80 mg per 24 hours
	Absent diural variation of plasma cortisol	8 A.M. plasma cortisol more than 50% of 8 A.M. value

ETIOLOGIC CLASSIFICATION OF CUSHING'S SYNDROME

	High Dose Dexa-methasone Response	*Metyrapone Response*	*ACTH Response*	*17-OH Excretion*	*17-KS Excretion*	*Other*
Pituitary lesion	50% fall urinary	Rise 17-OH steroids	Exaggerated High	High	High	? enlarged sella
Benign adenoma	None	None	Variable	High	Normal	
Adrenal carcinoma	None	None	None	High	Very high (4x)	Variable baseline
Ectopic ACTH syn.	None	Variable	Minimal	Very high (4x)	High	Variable baseline

CLINICAL FEATURES IN PRIMARY ALDOSTERONISM

Grouped Category	*Possible Presenting Signs or Symptoms*
Group I. Hypertension	Asymptomatic Symptomatic Visual disturbances Headache Cerebrovascular accident

Group II. Hypokalemia	Fatigue Paralysis Paresthesias Tetany Carbohydrate intolerance
Group III. Renal	Polyuria Polydipsia Nocturia

CLINICAL FEATURES IN ADDISON'S DISEASE

Grouped Category	*Possible Presenting Signs or Symptoms*
Group I. Asthenia	Decrease in strength and work capacity Irritability, drowsiness, and restlessness paralysis (hyperkalemic)
Group II. Cardiovascular	Hypotension, small heart
Group III. Gastrointestinal	Weight loss Food idiosyncrasy, poor appetite Disorder Anorexia, nausea, vomiting, diarrhea, abdominal pain
Group IV. Salt Wastage	Salt craving Muscle cramps Dizziness and syncope (hypotension)
Group V. Hypoglycemia	Coma
Group VI. Pigmentation	Recent scars, buccal mucosa, knuckles, elbows, palmar creases
Group VII. Miscellaneous	Loss of sex characteristics in female Vicarious calcification

PHEOCHROMOCYTOMA: PRESENTING FEATURES AND DIFFERENTIAL DIAGNOSIS

	Presenting Features	*Differential Diagnosis*
Group I.	Hypertension Episodic Paroxysmal dyspnea Persistent Cerebrovascular episodes	Essential hypertension Other causes of endocrine hypertension
Group II.	Spells Excessive perspiration Palpitations Pain (headache, angina, abdominal pain) Nevrousness and apprehension Paresthesia Pallor	Other causes of catecholamine release, e.g., hypoglycemia 5-hydroxy-tryptamine over-production Carcinoid Mastocytosis Menopausal symptoms Cervical spondylosis Horton's headaches Associated with use of monoamine oxidase inhibitors
Group III.	Metabolic Diabetes Loss of weight Fever	Diabetes mellitus Hyperthyroidism
Group IV.	Hypotension (rare) Hypovolemia Shock Polycythemia	Other causes of shock

DIAGNOSIS OF PHEOCHROMOCYTOMA

Critical Questions	*Special Tests*	*Comments*
Is the index of suspicion high?	Hypertension, Headache, Sweating, Palpitations	R/o reactive hypoglycemia

Are reliable metabolite assays abnormal? (Use two assays)	Metanephrine VMA (normal <6.8 mg/day) Free catecholamines	Values should be twice upper limit
Is a provocative test needed?	Measure urine after spontaneous epidode	
Provocative testing	Histamine (10 mg) Tyramine (500 mg) Glucagon (1 mg)	Dangerous in elderly Pretreatment with Dibenzyline if suspicion high; Using urinary metabo lite end point.
Alpha blockade	Phentolamine	Improved accuracy with insulin assays during i.v. glucose load
Localization	Oblique x-rays of spine Arteriography Surgical exploration	 Keep Phentolamine with patient

CLASSIFICATION OF DIABETES MELLITUS

Examples

A. *Primary*

Type 1 — Insulin-dependent diabetes mellitus (IDDM)

Type 2 — Non-insulin-dependent diabetes mellitus (NIDDM)

B. *Secondary to other pathology*

1. Pancreatic pathology — Pancreatitis
   - Haemochromatosis
   - Neoplastic disease
   - Pancreatectomy
   - Cystic fibrosis
2. Excess endogenous production of hormonal antagonists to insulin — Growth hormone (acromegaly)
   - Glucocorticoids (Cushing's syndrome)
   - Thyroid hormones (hyperthyroidism)
   - Catecholamines (phaeochromocytoma)
   - HPL (pregnancy)
   - Glucagon (glucagonoma)
   - Severe burns (glucagon, cortisol, cat echolamines)

	3. Medication with	Corticosteroids Thiazide diuretics Phenytoin
	4. Liver disease	
C.	*Associated with genetic syndromes*	DIDMOAD (i.e. diabetes insipidus, diabetes mellitus, optic atrophy, nerve deafness) Lipoatrophy Muscular dystrophies Friedreich's ataxia Down's syndrome Klinefelter's syndrome Turner's syndrome

CLINICAL FEATURES OF IDDM AND NIDDM

	IDDM	*NIDDM*
Genetic locus	Chr. 6	Chr. 11 (?)
Age at onset	< 40 years	>50 years
Duration of symptoms	Week	Months—years
Body weight	Normal or low	Obese
Ketonuria	Yes	No
Rapid death without treatment with insulin	Yes	No
Autoantibodies	Yes	No
Diabetic complication at diagnosis	No	10-20%
Family history of diabetes	No	Yes
Other autoimmune disease	Yes	No

THE SYNDROMES OF DIABETES MELLITUS

Low Output Failure	*High Output Failure*
Idiopathic islet cell failure Juvenile-onset diabetes mellitus Adult-onset diabetes mellitus (prone to develop ketoacidosis)	Maturity-onset diabetes mellitus Association with obesity Association with inappropirate insulin release and possible hypoglycemia Association with pregnancy

Islet cell destruction Pancreatitis Replacement of islet by iron, hemochromatosis (Cushing's syndrome, acromedaly)	High-output diabetes mellitus associated with other endocrinopathies High-output diabetes mellitus associated with uremia
Islet cell insufficiency Secondary to high output pancreatic failure Maturity-onset diabetes mellitus associated with obesity	Lipoatropic diabetes mellitus
Diabetes mellitus	associated with other endocrinopathies (e.g. Cushing's, acromegaly)
The insensitive islet	Maturity-onset diabetes mellitus with or without obesity (delayed insulin release)
The blocked islet	Inability of islet to release insulin after glucose, consequent upon Epinephrine (e.g., pheochromocytoma) Thiazide drugs, particularly diazoxide Diphenylhydantion Potassium depletion (aldosterone excess)

CLINICAL PRESENTATION OF DIABETES MELLITUS

Symptomless	Discovered on routine examination
Acute or Subacute Onset (typically <20 years to age)	Progressive loss of weight, despite hyperphagia Severe polyurea and polydipsia Diabetic acidosis and coma
Gradual Onset (usually >40 years of age)	Pruritis, generalized or perigenital Recurrent infections Polyuria and polydipsia Blurring of vision Frequently obese Confusion, obtundation, coma (glucose hyperosmolality syndrome) Postprandial hypoglycemia (uncommon)

Late Manifestations

Neuropathic	Sensory polyneuropathy (lower limbs)
	Single nerve lesions
	Autonomic neuropathy
	Amyotrophy
Vascular	Premature large vessel disease (atheroscleorsis)
	Small vessel disease (microangiopathy)
Renal	Glomerulosclerosis (nephrotic syndrome and uremia)
	Pyelonephritis
Ophthalmic	Diabetic retinopathy
	Cataract
	Glaucoma
Dermatologic	Necrobiosis lipoidica

COMMONLY USED DRUGS AFFECTING GLUCOSE TOLERANCE

Hyperglycemia	*Hypoglycemia*
Caffeine	Ethanol
Catecholamines	INH
Chlorpromazine	MAO inhibitors
Corticosteroids	PAS
Diphenylhydantoin	Phenylbutazone
Ethacrynic acid	Probenecid
Furosemide	Salicylates
Indomethacin	Sulfonamides
Marihuana	Thiouracil
Nicotine	
Oral contraceptives	
Thiazides	

CLUES TO COMPLICATIONS IN DIABETIC KETOACIDOSIS

Complication	*Clues*
Acute gastric dilatation	Vomiting of blood or coffee-ground material or erosive gastritis
Cerebral edema	Obtundation or coma with or without neurologic signs, especially if occurring after initial improvement
Hyperkalemia	Cardiac arrest
Hypoglycemia	Adrenergic or neurologic signs: rebound ketosis
Hypokalemia	Cardiac arrhythmias
Infection	Fever
Insulin resistance	Unremitting acidosis after 4-6 h or adequate therapy
Myocardial infarction	Chest pain, appearance of heart failure; appearance of hypotension despite adequate fluids
Mucormycosis	Facial pain, bloody nasal discharge, blackened nasal turbinates, blurred vision, proptosis
Respiratory distress syndrome	Hypoxemia in the absence of pneumonia, chronic pulmonary disease, or heart failure
Vascular thrombosis	Stroke like picture or signs of ischemia in nonnervous tissue

INSULIN-RESISTANT STATES

I. Prereceptor resistance
   A. Mutated insulins
   B. Anti-insulin antibodies

II. Receptor and postreceptor resistance
   A. Obesity
   B. Type A syndrome (absent or dysfunctional receptor)
   C. Type B syndrome (antibody to insulin receptor)
   D. Lipodystrophic states (partial or generalized)
   E. Leprechaunism

F. Ataxia-telangiectasia
G. Rabson-Mendenhall syndrome
H. Werson syndrome
I. Alstrom syndrome
J. Pineal hyperplasia syndrome

INDICATIONS FOR THERAPY IN DIABETES MELLITUS

Insulin

Diabctic acidosis
Juvenile diabetes mellitus
Diabetes mellitus secondary to known pancreatic disease
Symptomatic maturity-onset diabetes mellitus in whom dietary measures have failed
Maturity-onset diabetes mellitus
With subacute diabetic symptoms
During intercurrent infection
Pre-and postoperatively
Diabetes mellitus associated with known endocrine causes which are not remediable

Oral agents

Maturity-onset diabetes mellitus in whom measures have failed and insulin therapy is not feasible
Temporary diabetic state induced by glucocorticoid therapy

ONSET AND DURATION OF EFFECTS OF VARIOUS INSULINS

Onset	*Nomenclature*	*Remarks*
Early	*Crystalline zinc insulin* (CZI, regular crystalline, soluble) Maximal effect: 4-6 hours Duration: 6-8 hours	Compatible with all other insulins in mixture Used as supplement to other insulins; in acute illness; in examples of insulin resistance
	Semi-lente Maximal effect: 4-6 hours Duration: 12-16 hours	Action similar to CZI but duration is slightly longer Compatible with other members of lente family Not used intravenously

Intermediate	*Neutral-protamine* (Isophane, NPH) Maximal effect: 8-12 hours Duration: 12-18 hours	Most commonly used insulin for daytime needs May cause hypoglycemia in late afternoon, if taken in morning
	Globin Maximal effect: 6-10 hours Duration: 12-18 hours	Duration of action may be shorter than others in this group
	Lente Mixture of 3 semi-lente and 7 ultra-lente Mixture effect: 8-12 hours Duration: 18-24 hours	Quite similar to NPH Mixes with others of lente family Produces maximum effect in late afternoon, if taken in morning
Delayed	*Protamine zinc* (PZI) Maximal effect: 16-18 hours Duration: 24 hours or longer	Termination of action difficult to time Action of CZI delayed when mixed with this preparation (May lead to early morning hypoglycemia)
	Ultra-lente Maximal effect: 16-18 hours Duration: 30 hours or longer	Maximum action and duration of action similar PZI

MAJOR CAUSES OF FASTING HYPOGLYCEMIA

I. Conditions primarily due to underproduction of glucose
   A. Hormone deficiencies
      1. Hypopituitarism
      2. Adrenal insufficiency
      3. Catecholamine deficiency
      4. Glucagon deficiency
   B. Enzyme defects
      1. Glucose-6-phosphatase
      2. Liver phosphorylase
      3. Pyruvate carboxylase

4. Phosphoenolpyruvate carboxykinase
5. Fructose-1, 6-diphosphatase
6. Glycogen synthetase

C. Substrate deficiency
1. Ketotic hypoglycemia of infancy
2. Severe malnutriton, muscle wasting
3. Late pregnancy

D. Acquired liver disease
1. Hepatic congestion
2. Severe hepatitis
3. Cirrhosis
4. Uremia (probably multiple mechanisms)
5. Hypothermia

E. Drugs
1. Alcohol
2. Propranolol
3. Salicylates

II. Conditions primarily due to overuilization of glucose

A. Hyperinsulinism
1. Insulinoma
2. Exogenous insulin
3. Sulfonylureas
4. Immune disease with insulin or insulin receptor antibodies
5. Drugs: quinine in falciparum malaria, disopyramide, pentamidine
6. Endotoxic shock

B. Appropriate insulin levels
1. Extrapancreatic tumors
2. Systemic carnitine deficiency
3. Deficiency in enzymes of fat oxidation
4. 3-Hydroxy-3-methylglutaryl-CoA lyase deficiency
5. Cachexia with fat depletion

DIFFERENCES IN COMA DUE TO HYPOGLYCAEMIA AND KETOACIDOSIS IN IDDM

	Hypoglycaemic coma	*Coma with ketosis*
History	No food; too much insulin; unaccustomed exercise	Too little or no insulin; an infection; digestive disturbance
Onset	In good previous health; related to last insulin injection	Ill-health for several days
Symptoms	Hypoglycaemia; occasional vomiting from depot insulins	Of glycosuria and dehydration; abdominal pain and vomiting
Signs	Moist skin and tongue	Dry skin and tongue
	Full pulse	Weak pulse
	Normal or raised BP	Low blood pressure
	Shallow or normal breathing	Air hunger
	Brisk reflexes	Diminished reflexes
Urine	No ketonuria	Ketonuria
	No glycosuria, if bladder recently emptied	Glycosuria
Blood	Hypoglycaemia	Hyperglycaemia
	Normal plasma bicarbonate	Reduced plasma bicarbonate

HYPERPARATHYROIDISM

Primary	
Single adenoma (90%)	
Multiple adenoma (4%)	Serum calcium and PTH raised
Nodular hyperplasia (5%)	
Carcinoma (1%)	
Secondary	
Chronic renal failure	
Malabsorption	serum calcium low, PTH raised
Osteomalacia and rickets	
Tertiary	serum calcium and PTH raised

SERUM CONCENTRATIONS OF 1,25(OH)2D IN DISORDERS OF CALCIUM, PHOSPHORUS, AND BONE METABOLISM

Disease states	*Serum 1,25 (OH)2D*
Vitamin D deficiency	↓
Renal failure:	
GFR > (30 mL/min)/1.7 m^2	↓ or N
GFR < (30 mL/min)/1.7 m^2	
Hypoparathyroidism	↓ or N

Pseudohypoparathyroidism	↓ or N
Vitamin D—dependent rickets:	↓
Type I	↓ or N
Type II	↑ or N
X-linked vitamin D—resistant rickets	↓ or N
Tumor-induced osteomalacia	↓
Oncogenic hypercalcemia	↓
Some lymphomas	↑
Hyperparathyroidism	↑
Sarcoidosis, tuberculosis, silicosis	↑
Idiopathic, hypercalciuria	N or ↑
Williams' syndrome	↓
Vitamin D intoxication	↓ or N

* Serum 1,25(OH)2D concentrations are normal or elevated in occasional patients with biopsy-proven osteomalacia and undetectable or low circulating concentrations of 25(OH)D. these patients also have secondary hyperparathyroidism, and they may represent a partially treated state; if a small amount of vitamin D is obtained from the diet or generated in the skin in these patients, the vitamin is efficienty converted to 1,25(OH)2D. the net effect is low or undetectable circulating concentrations of 25(OH)D along with normal or elevated concentrations of 1,25(OH)2D. However, in extreme vitamin D deficiency, circulating concentrations of 1,25(OH)2D are low or undetectable.

Note: ↓ = decreased; N = Normal, ↑ = increased; GFR = glomerular filtration rate.

CLASSIFICATION OF PSEUDOHYPOPARATHYROIDISM (PHP) AND PSEUDOPSEUDOHYPOPARATHYROIDISM (PPHP)

Type	*Hypocalcemia, hyperphosphatemia*	*Response of Urinary cAMP to PTH*	*Serum PTH*	*G subunit deficiency*	*AHO*	*Resistance to hormones in addition to PTH*
PHP-Ia	Yes			Yes	Yes	Yes
PHP-Ib	Yes			No	No	No
PHP-II	Yes	Normal		No	No	No
PPHP	No	Normal	Normal	Yes	Yes	±

Note: ↓ = decreased; ↑ = increased; AHO = Albright's hereditary osteodystrophy

MALE HYPOGONADISM

Hypergonadotrophic Syndromes	
Klinefelter's Syndrome	Chromatin Positive Buccal Smear Classic XXY and mosaics poly X + Y
Reifenstein's	Hypospadias, gynecomastia
Sertoli-Cell-Only	Azospermia only
Anorchia	No testicles
"Male" Turner's Syndrome	Somatic features similar to those in females, XY and mosaics
XXY Syndrome	Increased height, acne, and often antisocial behavior
Post Orchitis Testicular Failure	Bacterial or viral Infection (gonorrhea, mumps, etc.) Posttraumatic Postirradiation
Myotonia Dystrophica	Present in about 80 percent
Adult Seminiferous Tubule Failure	
Adult Leydig Cell Failure	"Male climacteric"
Spinal Cord Damage	Traumatic or neoplasm
Hypogonadotrophic Syndromes	
Classic Eunuchoidism	LH-RH deficiency with resultant Low FSH and LH
Kallman's syndrome	Anosmia or hyposmia X-Linked dominant LH-RH
Fertile-Eunuch	? Hypothalamic etiology
Idiopathic Partial Hypopituitarism	Deficiency in LH, FSH, and GH
Panhypopituitarism	Prepubertal-Idiopathic pituitary dwarfism, primary benign and malignant or secondary neoplasms
Hypothalamic Dysfunction	Hypothalamic or adjacent neoplasms
Feminization	Estrogen producing adrenal or testicular neoplasm

GYNECOMASTIA

Adolescent Gynecomastia

Gynecomastia In Association With Gonadal Disorders

Klinefelter's syndrome

Reifenstein's syndrome

True hermaphrodite

Gynecomastia In Association With Systemic Disease

Cirrhosis of the liver

Bronchial carcinoma

Ulcerative colitis

High spinal cord lesions

Hodgkins disease

Bronchogenic carcinoma

Testicular tumors

Choricarcinoma, mixed cell, interstitial cell adenomas

Adrenal tunors

Femininizing adrenal carcinoma

Refeeding following mainutrition

Tuberculosis, diabetes, mellitus, cirrhosis

Thyroid dysfunction

Hyperthyroidism and rare hypothyroidism

Isolated Gynecomastia

Familial

Drug induced

Estrogens, testosterone, phenothiazine, meprobamate, hydrolyzine, reserpine, spironolactone, digitalis, marihuana

Mammary carcinoma

Renal failure on chronic hemodialysis

Idiopathic

Pseudogynecomastia of obesity

DIFFERENTIAL DIAGNOSIS-DIABETIC KETOACIDOSIS VERSUS HYPOGLYCEMIA

		Diabetic ketoacidosis	*Hypoglycemia*
1.	*Onset*	Show-few hrs. to 1-2 days	Rapid-minutes to few hrs.
2.	*Symptoms :*	Thirst	Hunger
		Headache	Fatigue
		Nausea	Confusion
		Vomiting	Irritability
		Abdominal pain	Inability ot concentrate
		Constipation	Headache

		Visual disturbances	Yawning
		Air hunger	Sweating
			Dizziness
			Blurred vision
			Paresthesia
3.	*Signs :*	Kussmaul respiration	Tremors
		Dehydration	Behavioural disturbances
		Flushed face	Pallor
		Rapid and thready pulse	Pulse full and bounding
		Hypothermia or sometimes fever	Ataxia
		Coma	Sweating
			Stupor Seizures (focal or generalized
			Coma

DIFFERENTIAL DIAGNOSIS OF SHORT STATURE

		Constitutional delay in growth	*Familial short stature*	*Pituitary dwarfism*	*Hypothyroidism*	*Turner syndrome*
1.	Family history	+ve	+ve	usually-ve	-ve	usually-ve
2.	Birth weight & height	N	↓	N	N	Slightly reduced
3.	Pattern of growth birth	Slow from birth months after birth	Slow from birth	Slow from a few	Slow from	Slow from birth
4.	Epiphyseal development	moderate but not progressive	almost normal	progressive retardation	marked retardation	within normla with variation

CLASSIFICATION OF ADRENAL DISORDERS

Congenital *Primary*	*Acquired* *Primary*
Inborn errors (enzyme deficiencies)	Adreno-cortical insufficiency
Congenital adrenal hyperplasia	Acute haemorrhage, infection, steroid suppression
Glucocorticoid deficiency	Chronic — 'Addison's syndrome
Mineralocorticoid deficiency	Adeno-cortical excess
Structural abnormalities	Glucocorticoids — Conn's syndrome
Congenital adrenal hypoplasia	Adrogens — premature adrenaarche, adenoma, carcinoma
Secondary	
Hypothalamic-pituitary insufficiency	

Mineralocorticoids —Conn's syndrome
Adreno-medullary excess
Phaeochromocytoma
Secondary
Hypothalamic—pituitary disease
Insufficiency
Excess-Cushing's syndrome

BIOCHEMICAL AND CLINICAL ABNORMALITIES IN THE VARIETIES OF CONGENITAL ADRENAL HYPERPLASIA

		Hormone status			*Genitalia*			
Enzyme defect	*ACTH*	*17-OH prog.*	*Cortisol*	*Aldo.*	*Male*	*Female*	*Salt balance*	*BP*
20-22 ↓	↑	↓	↓	↓	Amb	N	Loss ++	
3 ↓	↑	↓	↓	↓	Amb	± Viril	Loss +	
17	↑	↓	N or ↓	↓	Amb	N	Retention	↑
21	↑	↑	N or ↓	N or ↓	N	Viril	N or Loss ++	N or ↓
11	↑	↑	↓	↓	N	Viril	Retention	↑
18	N	N	N	↓	N	N	Loss +	↑

NAMED SIGNS (ORGAN-WISE)

PANCREAS

Grey- Guy's Sign: *Chronic relapsing pancreatitis*

... with the patient lying on the right side in the knee-chest position, palpation of the left subcostal region may evoke tenderness not otherwise found.

Trousseau's Sign: *Carcinoma of any part of pancreas.*

... thrombohlebitis migrans of the lower extremities (wandering thrombophlebitis is often the first striking sign of carcinoma pancreas).

Cullen's Sign: *Intraperitoneal haemorrhage* (especially in ruptured ectopic pregnancy)

... periumbilical darkening of the skin from blood.

ENDOCRINE

Orbital Signs of Primary thyrotoxicosis (Graves' Disease).

* **Stellwag's Sign** ... Widening of the palpebral fissure due to retraction of the upper eyelid — *Mild exophthalmos.*
* **Von Graefe's Sign** ... Persistent lagging of the upper eyelid — *Mild exophthalmos.*
* **Joffroy's Sign** ... Abscence of wrinkling of the forehead when the head is bent down and the patient looks upwards— *Moderate exophthalmos.*
* **Moebius's Sign:** Difficulty in convergence when the patient is asked to look at a near object — *Severe exophthalmos.*
* **Gifford's Sign** ... If the upper eyelid cannot be everted, or everted with difficulty, the exophthalmos is more likely to be due to thyrotoxicosis, whereas if the lid is everted easily it is more likely the presence of an intra-orbital mass.

Hypoparathyroidism

* **Chvostek's Sign** ... Tapping over the branches of the facial nerve at the angle of the jaw wall produces twitching at the corner of mouth, ala of nose and eyelids.
* **Trousseau's Sign** ... A sphygmomanometer cuff applied to the arm and inflated above the systolic BP for not more than 2 minutes will produce carpal spasm.

NAMES SYNDROMES

PANCREAS

* **WDHA Syndrome** : *Pancreatic cholera* (Water Diarrhoea, Hypokalemia, & Achlorhydria)

... caused by non-b islet cell tumour of the pancreas that secretes VIP (Vasoactive Intestinal Polypeptide) and histidine isoleucine- characterized by profuse watery diarrhoea, massive faecal loss of postassium, low serum potassium and extreme weakness. Gastric acid secretion is usually low or absent.

---

* **Zollinger-Ellison Syndrome :** *ZES type* I (rare) ... antral G-cell hyperplasia, hyper gastrinaemia and chronic peptic ulceration. *ZES type II* (due to ulcerogenic, non-b-islet-cell tumour or diffuse hyperplasia of islet cells secretes gastrin and is usually found in the tail of pancreas) ... intractable peptic ulceration (jejunum), hypergastrinaemiawith massive acid hypersecretion of upto 500 ml per hour, & diarrhoea, steatorrhoea or hypokalaemia.

  Treatment : ZES type I — partial gastrectomy. *ZES Type II* — if tumour - H2 receptor antagonist; if medical therapy fails ... Total gastrectomy.

THE ENDOCRINES

* ***Pendred's Syndrome*** ... Goitre is associated with congenital deafness (due to deficiency of peroxidase).
* **Sheehan's Syndrome** ... Simmond's disease (postpartum pituitary necrosis).
* **Conn's Syndrome** ... Primary aldosteronism.
* **Cushing's Syndrome** ... Post pubertal or adult hypercoticism.
* **Nelson's Syndrome** ... Hyperpigmentation & pituitary enlargement occurs in cases after bilateral adrenalectomy (in 20% cases).
* **Adrenogenital Syndrome** ... Adrenal androgen hypersecretion.
  * *Multiple Endocrine Neoplasia (MEN)*

    In the commoner type (Type I)

MEN 1... formerly known as *the pluriglandular syndrome,* the fol lowing abnomrmalities may be found:

Hyperparathyroidism (usually chief cell hyperplasia)

Pituirary tumour (acidophil or chromophobe adenomas)

Adrenal cortical adenomas (rarely)

Thyroid tumours (rarely)

This disorder may be familial, inherited as an autosomal dominant.

Multiple endocrine neoplasia (Type 2)

MEN 2... formerly known as *Sipple's syndrome,* may also be familial. Patients have one or more of the following :

Medullary carcinoma of the thyroid.
Phaeochromocytoma
Neurofibromatosis
Hyperparathyroidism
Cushing's syndrome (rarely)

* ***Familial Medullary Carcinoma syndrome:***
(MEN type II).
MEN II A : is more common type and it consists of multicentric medullary carcinoma or C-cel hyperplasia, phaeochromocytomas or adrenal medullary hyperplasia, and hyperpara thyroidism...
MEN II B : consists of Medullary carcinoma; phaeochromocytomas and mucosal neuromas of the lips, tongue, or conjunctiva; ganglioneuromas of the bowel; a typical appearance; and a Marfan like habitus.

COMPARISON OF THE THREE COMMON METHODS OF TREATMENT OF HYPERTHYROIDISM

	Method	*Action*	*Advantage*	*Disadvantage*
1.	Anti-thyroid drugs	Block thyroid hormone synthesis	1. Avoids surgery and irradiation	1. High incidence of drug reaction, action, blood dyscrasias, skin reaction 2. Frequent visits to physician necesary 3. Recurrence rate high when therapy discontinued.
II.	Surgery	Removal of functioning tissue	1. Most rapid method of permanent control 2. Avoids irradiation	1. Complications of surgery : a. Damage to recurrent laryngeal nerves b. Damage to parathyroid glands (1%) c. Wound complications d. Permanent hypothryoidism (30%)
III.	I^{131}	Radioactive destruction of thyroid cells	1. Avoids surgery 2. Permanent control 3. Avoids drugs reaction	1. Danger of irradiation 2. Hypothyroidism rate is high, 50% or more in 10 years; 3. Often treatment period is lengthy (up to 2 yeas) 4. Contraindicated in pregnancy and the very young

IMPORTANT DIAGNOSTIC THYROID TESTS

Test	*Normal values*	*Theory*	*Comments*
Serum thyroxine	4 to 11 µg%	Measures total thyroxine in serum	Neither inorganic nor organic iodides interfere: increased serum proteins elevate values; serum proteins depress values.
Radioactive Iodine uptake	15% to 40% 4 and 24 hr.	Measures amount and rate that thyroid takes up I131 in 4 and 24 hr	Most reliable test; not used during pregnancy; I2 and antithyroid drugs will block this test
T3 uptake test	25% to 35%	Measures excess radioactive T3 that becomes absorbed on resin; in toxic patients the protein; in toxic patients "saturated", thus radioactive T3 will be absorbed on resins	Radioactive T3 is incubated with patient's blood in vitro; can be used in pregnancy; not affected by I2 or antithyroid drugs; thus can be used to check patients treated iwth these drugs; low-serum proteins cause falsely increased values; increasd serum proteins cause falsely depressed values.
Scintiscan	Normal glands show an even distribution of I131 throughout gland	I131 map of thyroid	Cysts, nodules, and cancer may be "cold", little help in picking out malignant nodules, one definite asset is recording thyroid metatases to other areas (neck, bones, etc.)
Werner's test	4 and 24 hr. I131 uptake is depressed by 50% (after suppression with 5-day course of T3)	The pituitary-thyroid axis is tested by oral exogenous T3 to suppress TSH; normal patients will suppress by 50% toxic patients do not	Very useful in determining the borderline hyperthyroid patients, when other laboratory values are equivocal
BMR	± 15%	Measures O2 consumption	Inaccurate; false values in anxiety, starvation, tumors metabolic defects, different body builds
PBI	4 to 8 µg%	Direct measure of iodine attached to protein (thyroglobulin)	Extremely sensitive; any intake of iodides will falsely elevate values; values after myelography or bronchography are elevated almost indefinitely elevated in pregnancy depressed with diuretics.

FUNCTIONALLY BASED CLASSIFICATION OF HYPOCALCEMIA (EXCLUDING NEONATAL CONDITIONS)

I. PTH absent
   - A. Hereditary hypoparathyroidism
   - B. Acquired hypoparathyroidism
   - C. Hypomagnesemia

II. PTH ineffective
   - A. Chronic renal failure
   - B. Active vitamin D lacking

1. ↓ dietary intake or sunlight
2. Defective metabolism:
Anticonvulsant therapy
vitamin D—dependent rickets type I

C. Active vitamin D ineffective
1. Intestinal malabsorption
2. Vitamin D—dependent rickets type II

D. Pseudohypoparathyroidism

III. PTH overwhelmed

A. Severe, acute hyperphosphatemia
1. Tumor lysis
2. Acute renal failure
3. Rhabdomyolysis

B. Osteitis fibrosa after parathyroidectomy

CAUSES OF HYPOPHOSPHATEMIA

I. *Decreased dietary intake*

II. *Decreased intestinal absorption*

A. Vitamin D deficiency
B. Malabsorption
C. Steatorrhea
D. Secretory diarrhea
E. Vomiting

III. *Shifts from serum into cells*

A. Respiratory alkalosis
1. Sepsis

2.Glucagon

3. Epinephrine
4. Androgens
5. Cortisol
6. Anovulatory hormones

C. Nutrient effects
1. Glucose
2. Fructose
3. Glycerol
4. Lactate

5. Amino acids
6. Xylitol

D. Cellular uptake syndromes
1. Recovery from hypothermia
2. Burkitt's lymphoma
3. Histiocytic lymphoma
4. Acute myelomonocytic leukemia
5. Acute myelogenous leukemia
6. Treatment of pernicious anemia
7. Hungry bone syndrome
a. Following parathyroidectomy
b. Acute leukemia

IV. *Increased excretion into the urine*
A. Hyperparathyroidism
B. Renal tubular defects
1. Renal rickets
2. Polyostotic fibrous dysplasia
3. Postrenal transplantation
4. Oncogenic osteomalacia
C. Aldosteronism
D. Licorice ingestion
E. Volume expansion
F. Inappropriate secretion of vasopressin
G. Mineralocorticoid administration
H. Glucocorticoid therapy
I. Diuretics

CAUSES OF HYPOMAGNESEMIA

I. Primary nutritional disturbances
A. Inadequate intake
B. Total parenteral nutrition
C. Refeeding syndrome

II. Gastrointestinal disorders
   A. Specific absorptive defects
   B. Malabsorption syndromes
      1. Enteric fistulas
      2. Nontropical sprue
      3. Whipple disease
      4. Intestinal lymphoma
      5. Chronic pancreatic insufficiency
      6. Biliary diversion
      7. Giardiasis
      8. Short bowel syndrome
   C. Prolonged diarrhea
   D. Prolonged nasogastric suction
   E. Pancreatitis
III. Endocrine disorders
   A. Hyperparathyroidism
   B. Hypoparathyroidism
   C. Hyperthyroidism
   D. Primary hyperaldosteronism
   E. Bartter's syndrome
   F. Diabetic ketoacidosis
   G. Alcoholic ketoacidosis
   I. Syndrome of inappropriate secretion of anti-diuretic hormone
   J. "Hungry bones" syndrome after parathyroidectomy
IV. Chronic alcoholis; alcoholic withdrawal
V. Increased renal excretion
   A. Idiopathic
   B. Following renal transplantation

C. Cisplatin therapy

D. Aminoglycoside therapy

E. Amphotericin B therapy

F. Diuretics

1. Furosemide
2. Ethacrynic acid
3. Acetazolamide
4. Thiazides
5. Chlorthalidone
6. Osmotic agents

G. Recovery phase of acute tubular necrosis

ORIGINAL SOLVED MCQ's IN DM ENDOCRINOLOGY

1. **Which of the following hormones is not secreted by the adenohypophysis :**
   A. ADH B. ACTH
   C. TSH D. FSH

2. **The hormone with the shortest half life in the blood stream in the following list is :**
   A. Epinephrine B. Acetylcholine
   C. Insulin D. T3

3. **Following are local hormones except :**
   A. Insulin B. Heparin
   C. Bradykinin D. Acetyl choline

4. **Hormone secreted by hypothalamus is :**
   A. Somatastatin B. Somatatrophin
   C. Gonadotrophan D. Luleotrophin

5. **Alpha and beta types of receptors are used to explai pharmacological actions of :**
   A. Cholinergic B. Adrenergic
   C. Muscarinic D. Nicotinic

6. **What detemines whether norepinephrine circulating in the bod fluids will be excitatory of inhibitory in a particular organ?**
   A. The nature of the receptor in the cells of the oxgen
   B. The intensity of nerve stimulation of the oxgen
   C. The chemical changes that occur in the norepinephrine before excites the cells
   D. The position on the cells where norepinephrine is secreted by th nerve endings

7. **Enzyme involved in acetylcholine synthesis is :**
   A. Choline acetyl transferase
   B. Choline esterase
   C. Pseudo cholinesterase
   D. Glycine

Ans. 1. A 2. B 3. A 4. A 5. B 6. A 7. A

8. The secretion of aldosterone is caused by :

A. Angiotensin B. ACTH
C. Epinephrine D. Insulin

9. Which of the following decreases insulin secretion :

A. Growth hormone B. Glucocorticoids
C. Epinephrine D. Glucose

10. Abnormal catecholamine metabolism is seen in :

A. Neuroblastoma B. Wilms tumo
C. Lympho sarcoma D. Ewings tumour

11. Experimental diabetes is caused by :

A. Alloxan B. PgE1
C. Radioactive yitrium D. Gold chloride

12. Which of the following statements is not correct? Release of acetylcholine at the neuromuscular junca-tion :

A. Produces an end-plate potential
B. Increase sodium movement into the muscle cell
C. Always causes the muscle fiber to contract
D. Is followed by rapid destruction of acetylcholine

13. Which of the following does not act at receptors :

A. TRH B. Thyroxine
C. Insulin D. Epinephr

14. Simmond's disease is characterized by all except :

A. Infertility B. Increase BMR
C. Increase Immunity D. Polyurea

15. Uterine contracility is increased by hormone :

A. Progesterone B. LH
C. FSH D. Oestrogen

16. Gluconeogenesis requires the action of :

A. Growth hormone B. Insulin
C. Estradiol D. Calcitoni

17. The only hormone for which no stimulatory factor has been isolated is :

A. Growth hormon B. Gonadotropin
C. Thyroxine D. Prolactin

18. Which of the following is not caused by estrogen ?

A. ↓ serum Alkaline phosphatase
B. ↑ Blood sugar
C. ↓ Folate level
D. ↑ HDL

Ans.	8. A	9. C	10. A	11. A	12. C	13. B
	14. B	15. D	16. A	17. D	18. B	

19. Menopausal hot flushes is due to :

A. FSH surge B. LH surge

C. Decreased estrogen D. Decreased progesterone

20. Increase in Insulin receptors is seen in:

A. Acromegaly B. Starvation

C. Obesity D. Diabetes

21. Which neurotransmitter controls secretion of Prolactin?

A. Dopamine B. Serotonin

C. Somatostatin D. GABA

22. Urine osmolality in Diabetes insipidus is :

A. 150 mmol/L B. 300 mmol/L

C. 600 mmol/L D. 900 mmol/L

23. Following are changes seen in SIADH except :

A. Low plasma osmolality B. Low urine osmolality

C. Hyponatremia D. Edema

24. Insulin promotes transport of glucose in which of these ?

A. Adipose tissue B. RBC

C. Muscles D. Hepatocytes

25. Steroids are synthesized by :

A. Smooth ER B. Rough ER

C. Mitochondria D. Lysosomes

26. Deficient adrenal function leads to rise in blood :

A. Sodium B. Glucose

C. Pressure D. Potassium

27. A patient with a secreting tumour of adrenal medulla (phaeochromocytoma) typically has :

A. Raised blood pressure transient or constant

B. A fine tremor of extended hand

C. Lowering of blood pressure when alpha adrenoceptor antagonist is given

D. Increase in BMR

E. All of the above

28. Growth hormone secretion is increased in normal person in all of the following except :

A. Exercise B. Hyperglycemia

C. Infusion of Levodopa D. Infusion of Arginine

29. The likelihood of developing tetany is increased when :

A. Plasma HCO_3 rises

B. Plasma magnesium rises

C. Respiratory failure develops

D. Anterior pituitary removed

Ans.					
19. B	20. B	21. A	22. B	23. B	24. D
25. A	26. D	27. E	28. B	29. A	

30. TSH is secreted at a higher rate :

A. After removal of one lobe of thyroid
B. In warm adapted than in cold adapted persons
C. When BMR falls
D. During physical injury and emotional stress

31. In the absence of ADH (Anti-dieuritic Hormone) :

A. There would not be any water absorption in renal tubules
B. Facultative water absorption is deficient
C. Facultative water absorption is increased
D. Obligatory water absorption is increased

32. Sertoli cells secrete :

A. Testosterone
B. Androstenedione
C. PG E2
D. Estrogens

33. Calcium metabolism is mainly dependent on :

A. Calcitonin
B. Parathormone
C. Thyroxine
D. Growth hormone

34. Activation of renin-angiotensin mechnism result in the following except :

A. Aldosterone secretion
B. Increased arteriolar tone
C. Decrease in renal sodium excretion
D. Decrease in blood volume

35. Production of aldosterone under normal conditions will be influenced by all except :

A. Blood sodium level
B. Blood angiotensin level
C. Crystalloid osmotic pattern of blood
D. ACT

36. Which of the following is not true about calcium metabolism :

A. Phytates in diet increase absorption
B. Dihydroxycholecalciferol increases absorption
C. High protein diet increases absorption
D. 40% of total calcium is in ionized form

37. Aldosterone secretion is regulated by following except :

A. ACTH
B. Calcium
C. Blood volume
D. Potassium

38. Menopause is caused due to :

A. Endometrium becomes insensitive to oestrogen & progesterone
B. Ovary does not produce oestrogen & progesterone
C. Pituitary
D. Hypothalamus

Ans.						
	30. A	31. B	32. D	33. B	34. D	35. D
	36. A	37. B	38. B			

39. **Thyroxin causes following except :**
A. Increased BMR
B. Increased cholesterol
C. Increased Beta-I-receptors
D. Increased heat production

40. **Hyperthyroidsm is associated with :**
A. Positive nitrogen balance
B. A decreased urinary excretion of calcium
C. A rise in level of plasma protein which binds thyroxine
D. Certain feature due to excessive beta adrenergic stimulation

41. **Hyperglycemia is associated with :**
A. ↓ Insulin secretion
B. ↑ Glucagon secretion
C. ↑ Insulin and glucagon secretion
D. A and B

42. **The thyroid hormone stored in the lumen of follicles is in the form of :**
A. Free T3
B. Free T4
C. Attached to thyroglobulin
D. Attached to thyroid binding globulin

43. **All of the following pituitary hormones are derived from basophilic and acidophilic cells except :**
A. GH
B. ACTH
C. PIH
D. FSH

44. **All of the following are true about insulin except :**
A. Glucose is absorbed from renal tubules
B. Short polypeptide with C-chain
C. Proinsulin is coiled and cross linked by disulfide bonds
D. Proinsulin is inactive

45. **Cortisol :**
A. Secretion increases following injury
B. Favours protein synthesis
C. Enhances effects of antigen-antibody reactions
D. Tends to lower blood pressure

46. **Aldosteronism is associated with :**
A. Oedema
B. Retention of sodium
C. Retention of potassium
D. Hypotension

47. **Calcitonin is responsible for :**
A. Increasing the plasma Ca^{++} level
B. Decreasing the plasma Ca^{++} level

Ans.	39. B	40. D	41. D	42. C	43. C	44. A
	45. A	46. B	47. B			

C. Increasing parathormone level
D. Decreasing thyroxine level

48. Regarding Myxoedema the following are true except :
A. Swollen, Oedematous look of the face
B. Impotency, amenorrhoea etc
C. B.M.R. increased by 30-45%
D. Dullness, loss of memory

49. The following features are found in hyperthroidism except :
A. Enlarged thyroid
B. Exophthalmos
C. Decreased body weight
D. Decreased B.M.R.

50. Regarding parathyroid the following statements are true except :
A. It regulates Ca and P metabolism
B. Controls the balance of inorganic ions in blood
C. It is not essential for life
D. Its cellular effects are mediated through Cyclic AMP

51. In Cushing syndrome the following features are found except :
A. Rapidly increasing adiposity
B. Polycythaemia
C. Hypotension
D. Impotence with atrophy of testis

52. Progesterone is secreted by the following except :
A. Corpus luteum
B. Placenta
C. Adrenal cortex
D. Testis

53. Epinephrine predominantly causes :
A. Glycogenolysis
B. Gluconeogenesis
C. Glycolysis
D. Glycogen storage

54. Estrogens in the post menopausal period is metabolized mostly into :
A. Estriol
B. Estrone
C. Estradiol
D. Androstenedione

55. FSH is secreted by :
A. Chromophobes
B. Acidophils
C. Basophils
D. Theca internal cells

56. Transection of the Pituitary stalk leads to increase in :
A. Growth Hormone
B. TSH
C. Prolactin
D. ACTH

57. Anabolic action on proteins is mediated by :
A. Growth hormone
B. Insulin
C. ACTH
D. Testosterone

Ans.	48. C	49. D	50. C	51. C	52. D	53. A
	54. B	55. C	56. C	57. D		

58. **Following are true of insulin except :**
A. Glycopeptide
B. Secreted by Beta cells
C. Causes lipogenesis
D. Promotes glycogenesis

59. **Estrogens acts on :**
A. Cell membrane
B. Nucleus
C. Mitochondria
D. Cytoplasmic receptor

60. **In diabetic ketosis, there is a decreased metabolic breakdown of :**
A. Fat
B. Protein
C. Glucose
D. Glycogen liver

Match the following :
A. Cortisol
B. Androgen
C. Aldosteone
D. Norepinephrine

61. **Zona glomerulosa :**
62. **Zona relicularis :**
63. **Zona fasciculata :**
64. **Adrenal medulla :**

65. **Peak testosterone levels are seen at about :**
A. 7-8 PM
B. 2 AM
C. 7-8 AM
D. 12 PM

66. **Following are the effects of testosterone except :**
B. Calcium retention
C. Increased Total quantity of bone matrix
D. Increased BMR

67. **Amino acid sequence of human insulin differs from porcine insulin in :**
A. 1 amino acid
B. 3 amino acids
C. 5 amino acids
D. None of the above

68. **Which of the following arterioles is least sensitive to epinephrine :**
A. Skeletal muscle arteriole
B. Cerebral
C. Cutaneous
D. Afferent renal

69. **The following hormones increase the level of intra-cellu-lar cAMP except :**
A. Vasopressin
B. Glucagon
C. Parathyroid hormone
D. Somatostatin

70. **Which of the following G protein is associated with receptors for norepinephrine :**
A. Gt1
B. Gi1
C. Gt2
D. Go

72. **The size and number of inclusions in the type II alveolar epithelial cells producing surfactant are increased by :**
A. Growth hormone
B. Androgens
C. Thyroxine
D. Insulin

Ans.						
	58. A	59. B	60. C	61. C	62. B	63. A
	64. D	65. C	66. A	67. A	68. B	69. D
	70. C	71. B	72. C			

73. The following in true about carbonic anhydrase except :

A. A protein with a molecular weight of 30,000

B. Contains an item of copper in each molecule

C. Inhibited by cyanide, azide and sulfide

D. Sulfonamides also inhibit this enzyme

74. Islet cells of Pancreas secrete all of the following except :

A. Somatostatin

B. Gastrin

C. VIP

D. Pancreozymin

75. Pheochromocytomas predominantly secrete :

A. Epinephrine

B. Norepinephrine

C. 5-HT

D. Renin

76. Which of the following responses is not initiated by the stimulation of adrenergic sympathetic neurons ?

A. Hepatic glycogenolysis

B. Skeletal muscle vasoconstriction

C. Ventricular force increase

D. Ventricular conduction time increase

E. Contraction of pyloric sphincter of stomach

77. An animal deprived of its adrenal glands :

A. Loses most of its reactions due to increased sym-pathetic activity, because of the lack of circulating epinephrine

B. Can still develop tachycardia and sympathetic hypertension in response to exercise

C. Has a much greater rate of glycogenolysis

D. Usually is hyperglycemic during fasting periods

78. When a patient is treated with aldosteone antagonist there is likely to be a fall in ?

A. Urine volume

B. Plasma postassium level

C. Blood volume

D. Blood viscosity

79. Increased release of aldosterone from adrenal cortex is not a feature in :

A. Increased arterial pressure

B. Hyponatremia

C. Hyperkalemia

D. Epinephrine and norepinephrine

80. If there is a decrease in extracellular fluid volume, the body may respond by increasing the secretion of :

A. Epinephrine

B. Aldosterone

C. Epinephrine and aldosterone

D. Epinephrine, aldosterone and A.D.H.

Ans.	**73. B**	**74. D**	**75. A**	**76. D**	**77. B**	**78. C**
	79. A	**80. D**				

81. **True about gastrin is :**
   A. A peptide hormone
   B. An analogue of Pentagastrin which decreases secretion of HCl
   C. Secreted with HCl from parietal cells
   D. Increased in Zollinger Ellison syndrome

82. **Somogyl phenomenon is :**
   A. Hypoglycemia followed by hyperglycemia
   B. Hypoglycemia followed by hypoglycemia
   C. Glycosuria with normal blood sugar
   D. Reactive hyperglycemia

83. **Pain producing substance is :**
   A. Serotonin B. Substance P
   C. Histamine D. Acetylcholine

84. **Cyclic AMP serves as second messenger in the secre-tion of all except :**
   A. FSH B. Estrogen
   C. Glucagon D. Epinephrine

85. **Function of Leutenizing hormone is :**
   A. Follicle maturation and ovulation
   B. Milk secretion
   C. Causes progesterone secretion during ovulation
   D. Maintain placenta

86. **Precursor of testesterone is :**
   A. Methyl testeterone B. Pregnenalone
   C. Aldosteone D. Cortisone

87. **Metyrapone is useful in congenital hyperplasia because it inhibits :**
   A. 17-alpha hydroxylase B. 21-alpha hydroxylase
   C. 11-beta hydroxylase D. Desmolase

88. **FSH and ICSH are secreted by :**
   A. Adenohypophysis B. Hypothalamus
   C. Ovaries D. Placenta

89. **Position of estradiol/OH is at :**
   A. C3 & C17 B. C & C
   C. C & C D. C & C

90. **Hormones secreted by anterior pituitary lobe is/are :**
   A. GH B. Prolactin
   C. TSH D. All

91. **Function of acini in thyroid gland is synthesis of :**
   A. Tyrosine B. Thyroxine
   C. Mucus D. TSH

Ans.	81. D	82. A	83. B	84. B	85. A	86. B
	87. C	88. A	89. A	90. D	91. B	

92. Which of the following does not have natriuretic actions :

A. Aldosterone B. Natriuretic peptide
C. Angiotensin D. Prednisolone

93. The hormone responsible for increased body temperature after ovulation is :

A. Lutenizing hormone B. Progesterone
C. Increased estrogen D. Androgens

94. Secretion of estriol during pregnancy :

A. Is independent on both a viable fetus and a functioning placenta
B. Is largely produced by the maternal ovaries
C. Is not dependent on a viable fetus
D. Is lower than the secretion rate of etriol is non-pregnancy body

95. Which is not formed in tryptophan metabolism :

A. Melatonin B. Dopamine
C. Serotonin D. Epinephrine

96. Beta endorphins are found in high concentration in :

A. Substantia gelatinosa B. Post pituitary
C. Spinal cord D. Medulla

97. Most potent vasopressor is :

A. Angiotensin II B. Renin
C. Aldosterone D. Cortisol

98. Levels of which of the following hormones are increased in post menopausal women :

A. Estrogen B. FSH
C. Progesteron D. Cortisone

99. Blockage of the hypothalamic-hypophyseal venous portal system would be expected to cause increased secretion of :

A. Growth hormone
B. Adrenocorticotropic hormone
C. Thyroid-stimulating hormone
D. Prolactin

100. High plasma levels of thyroxine can lead to all of the following except :

A. Increased cardiac output
B. Increased plasma triglyceride concentration
C. Increased heart rate
D. Decreased body weight

Ans.	92. A	93. B	94. A	95. B	96. A	97. A
	98. B	99. D	100. B			

101. **Thyroid-stimulating hormone stimulates thyroid function in many ways, but it does not increase :**
A. Synthesis of thyroxine-binding globulin
B. Rate of synthesis of thyroglobulin
C. Iodine uptake from the blood
D. Iodination of tyrosine

102. **Cortisol can cause all of the following except :**
A. Inflammation to be suppressed
B. Fat to be used for energy
C. Lysosomal membranes to become unstable
D. The blood glucose concentration to increase

103. **Growth hormone increases all of the following except :**
A. Blood glucose concentration
B. Blood free fatty acid concentration
C. Protein synthesis
D. None of the above

104. **All of the following hormones mediate their major effects without actually entering the target cell except :**
A. Cortisol
B. Insulin
C. Growth hormone
D. Glucagon

105. **Increased plasma parathyroid hormone concentra-tion tends to increase all of the following except :**
A. Number of active osteoclasts
B. Extracellular phosphate concentration
C. Absorption of calcium from the gastrointestinal tract
D. Absorption of calcium from the renal tubules

106. **The active form of Vitamin D is :**
A. Calcitonin
B. 1, 25 dihydroxycholecalciferol
C. Parathyroid hormone
D. Cholecalciferol

107. **Important effects of testosterone include all of the following except :**
A. Formation of the fetal penis
B. Descent of the testes into the scrotum
C. Increased muscle development
D. Initiation of ejaculation

108. **Synthesis of testosterone is controlled by :**
A. LH
B. LHRH
C. FSH
D. TSH

Ans.					
101. A	**102. C**	**103. D**	**104. A**	**105. B**	**106. B**
107. D	**108. A**				

109. Cortisol increases the blood glucose concentration either directly or indirectly by :

A. Decreasing glucose uptake by the cells
B. Decreasing the rate of gluconeogenesis
C. Decreasing the rate of glucose utilization by the cells
D. Inhibiting hormone-sensitive lipase

110. The principal estrogen found in the urine of pregnant women is :

A. Estriol
B. Estrone
C. Beta-estradiol
D. Pregnanediol

111. Which of the following statements about thyroxine is false ?

A. Its production requires the amino acids tyrosine
B. Its effect is slower in onset and longer in duration than that of triiodothyronine (T3)
C. It increases cerebral metabolic oxygen consumption
D. It is essential for the production of erythrocytes

112. Which of the following statements about androgens is false ?

A. They are formed by seminiferous tubules of the testis
B. they are formed in greater quantities in foetal life (in the male foetus) than in childhood
C. Are secreted in small amounts in normal audlt femlaes
D. Their concentration in blood decreases after the age of 30 in me

113. Which of the following statements about calcitonin is false ?

A. It reduces the number and activity of osteoclasts
B. It reduces the renal tubular absorption of calcium
C. It reduces the renal tubular absorption of phosphate
D. When present in excess, it commonly causes tetany

114. In which of the following organ, glucose uptake depends on insulin :

A. Renal epithelium
B. Heart
C. Brain
D. Intestinal epithelium

115. Vitamin D deficiency leads to :

A. Decreased calcium absorption by renal tubules
B. Decreased calcium absorption by intestine
C. Increased phsophate excretion by renal tubules
D. None of the above

116. The following substances cross blood brain barrier :

A. Insulin
B. Testosterone
C. Glucose
D. All of the above

Ans.	**109. C**	**110. A**	**111. C**	**112. A**	**113. D**	**114. B**
	115. B	**116. C**				

117. In the female rat, selective neutralization of follicle-stimulating hormone with anti-FSH antibodies :

A. Increases estrogen and progesterone secretion by the corpus luteum
B. Prevents early uniting of the epiphyses
C. Prevents early follicular growth
D. Suppresses the secretion of hypothalamic releasing factors

118. Spontaneous hypoglycemia may be caused by :

A. Glucagonoma
B. Chronic Pancreatitis
C. Cushing's syndrome
D. Hepatocellular carcinoma

119. `C' cells are present in :

A. Thyroid
B. Adrenal
C. Parathyroid
D. Pituitary

120. Stimulation of both glucocorticoid and mineralocorticoid secretion is seen with :

A. Anxiety
B. Exercise
C. Hyperkalemia
D. Low sodium diet

121. After drinking a large amount of hypotonic fluid and after absorption of the fluid from the gut into the blood, which of the following changes would you expect :

A. Increased secretion of antidiuretic hormone
B. A decrease in distal tubular permeability to water
C. A marked decrease in glomerular filtration rate
D. A marked increase in sodium excretion

122. Overall regulating organ for neuroendocrinal system is :

A. Hypothalamus
B. Pituitary
C. Reticulo-endothelial system
D. Pineal gland

123. Calcitonin is produced by:

A. Thyroid
B. Parathyroid
C. Thymus
D. Kidney

124. Maximum production of HCG occurs during :

A. First trimester
B. Second trimester
C. Third trimester
D. Implantation

125. Melatonin is secreted by :

A. Hypothalamus
B. Adrenal cortex
C. Pineal gland
D. Melanocytes

126. The excretion of estrogens and progesterone are through :

A. Bile
B. Sweat
C. Urine
D. Faeces

Ans.	117. C	118. B	119. A	120. A	121. B	122. A
	123. A	124. A	125. C	126. C		

127. In the testes, the cells that secrete testosterone are :

A. Germinal epithelium B. Leydig cells
C. Sertoli cells D. Sperm cells

128. Estrogen secretion by the ovary is influence of the following except :

A. Follicle stimulatory hormone
B. Luteinizing hormone
C. Sympathetic nerve activity
D. Progesteone

129. ACTH is most effective in stimulating the secretion of :

A. Hydrocortisone
B. Cortisone
C. Adrenal androgenic hormones
D. Aldosterone

130. Luteal phase of menstrual cycle is characterized by :

A. A variable length
B. Secretion of oestogen
C. Low basal body temperature
D. Secretion on progesterone

131. Which of the following hormone acts by decreasing cAMP levels :

A. Epinephrine (Beta 1 receptors)
B. Dopamine (D2 receptors)
C. Glucagen
D. None of the above

132. Reverse T3 is :

A. Synthetic derivative
B. Isomerisation product of T1 and active
C. Isomerisation product of T3 and inactive
D. Reverse T1

133. Actions of insulin except :

A. Glycolysis B. Glycogenesis
C. Lipogenesis D. Gluconeogenesis

134. Dopamine is inhibitor of:

A. Prolactin B. Growth hormone
C. Oxytoein D. Epinephrine

135. Spermatogenic epithelium is maintained by :

A. Somatostatin B. TRH
C. FSH D. LH

136. Level of T3 indicates :

A. Metabolic state B. Thyroid state
C. Pituitary function state D. Not importan

Ans.	127. B	128. C	129. A	130. D	131. D	132. C
	133. D	134. A	135. C	136. C		

137. Gonadal function is regulated by :

A. Anterior hypothalamus B. Posterior hypothalamus
C. Anterior pituitary D. Posterior pituitary

138. The prohormone produced by the theca interna of the ovary is :

A. α 17- ketosteroid B. An estrogen
C. A dehydroepiandrosterone D. All of these

139. The hormone which diminishes the exceretion of magnesium is :

A. Antiduretic hormone (ADH) B. Parathormone (PTH)
C. Growth hormone (G.H.) D. Aldosterone

140. Every nucleated cell has one of the following proteins which is involved in transmission of the message of many hormones called :

A. Calcium binding protein B. Calmodulin
C. Apotransferrin D. Apoceruloplamin

141. A cortisol deficient individual :

A. Has reduced resistance to stress
B. Has increased ability to mobilize stored triglyceride
C. Has reduced sensitivity to insulin
D. Shows all of these

142. All of the following are the actions of glucocorticoids on blood cells except :

A. Decrease in the number of Eosinophils
B. Decrease in the number of Basophils
C. Increase in the number of lymphocytes
D. Increase in the number of neutrophils and platelets
E. Increase in the number of Red blood cells

143. Which of the following statements about progesterone is not true ?

A. It stimulates the development of lobules and alveoli in the breast
B. It increases the excitability of myometrium
C. It is thermogenic
D. It can prevent ovulation in large doses
E. In large doses it produces natriuresis

144. cAMP action mediates all except :

A. Glucagon B. FSH
C. LH D. Estrogen

145. Thyroxine is injected to rat A/E :

A. $\downarrow\downarrow$ lipolysis B. $\uparrow\uparrow$ O2 consumption
C. $\downarrow$ BMR D. $\uparrow$myocardial contractility

146. FSH is produced by :

A. Chromphobes B. Acidophils
C. Basophils D. All of the above

Ans.	137. C	138. D	139. D	140. A	141. D	142. C
	143. B	144. D	145. C	146. C		

147. A person who is on starvation for 5 days. Glucose is given for GTT will cause the following except : AI 2001

A. GH decrease
B. Decreased Insulin
C. Increase cortisol
D. Increased Insulin tolerance

148. Lack of which of the following hormone causes osteoporosis :

A. Oestrogen
B. Progesterone
C. Thyroxine
D. Testosterone

149. Which of the following feature is not seen in hypopituitary state :

A. Cachexia
B. Growth failure
C. Infertility
D. Increased sensitivity to insulin

150. Secretion does not increase in night :

A. Growth hormone
B. ACTH
C. Insulin
D. TSH

151. Thyroxine does not increase the metabolism in :

A. Heart
B. Liver
C. Pitutary
D. Kidney

152. Which is produced in Cushings syndrome in excess :

A. Epinephrine
B. Norepinephrine
C Cortisol
D. Dopa

153. On injecting, concentrated NaCl solution into the carotid artery, there was increased production of ADH. The source of it's secretion in the hypothalamus is in the :

A. Paraventricular nucleus
B. Supraoptic nucleus
C. Anterior nucleus
D. Ventromedial nucleus

154. FSH acts on :

A. Theca cell
B. Granulosa cell
C. Stromal cell
D. Interstitial cell

W.155. Following have both alpha and beta subunits except :

A. TSH
B. LH
C. FSH
D. HCG

156. The blood testis barrier is seen in :

A. Leydig cells
B. Spermatogonia
C. Sertoli cells
D. Spermatozoa

157. Which of the following is an endocrine organ :

A. Lamina dura
B. Small intestine
C. Ciliary body
D. Breast

Ans.	147. B	148. A	149. A	150. B	151. C	152. C
	153. B	154. B	155. NONE	156. C	157. B	

158. Steroid hormones are produced by all except :

A. Testis
B. Placenta
C. Ovaries
D. Adrenal Medulla

159. Somatostatin Inhibits all except :

A. GH
B. ACTH
C. TSH
D. Prolactin

160. Thyrotropin release is mainly dependent on :

A. Thyroid status
B. TIBG levels
C. Levels of thyroid hormones in blood
D. Catecholamine levels

161. Circadian rhythm of ACTH is controlled by :

A. Supraoptic nucleus of hypothalamus
B. Paraventricular nucleus of hypothalamus
C. Suprachiasmatic nucleus of hypothalamus
D. Lateral nucleus of hypothalamus

162. The laboratory report shows values of gonadotropin and ovarian hormones of the blood sample taken on day 20 of the menstrual cycle of a young woman. Whether her cycle was ovulatory or not may be validly assessed by the reported serum level of :

A. FSH
B. LH
C. Oestradiol
D. Progesterone

163. Even in the presence of vasopressin the greatest fraction of filtered water is reabsorbed in which part of the nephron :

A. Proximal tubule
B. Distal tubule
C. Loop of Henle
D. Collecting duct

164. The hormone associated with cold adaptation is :

A Growth hormone.
B Thyroxine.
C Insulin.
D Melanocyle Stimulating Hormone.

165. In which of the following forms the Anti diuretic hormone (ADH) is circulated is plasma?

A. Bound to neurophysin - I
B. Bound to neurophysin - II
C. Bound to plasma albumin
D. Free form

166. Sertoli cells have receptors for?

A. Inhibin
B. Luteinising hormone
C. Follicle stimulating hormone
D. Melatonin

Ans.	158. D	159. D	160. C	161. C	162. D	163. A
	164. B	165. B	166. D			

167. Before the onset of puberty, the GnRH neurons are under the inhibitory control of ?

A. Glycine
B. Glutamate
C. Gamma amino butyric acid (GABA)
D. Beta-endorphin

168. The enzyme associated with the conversion of androgen to oestrogen in the growing ovarian follicle is?

A. Desmolase B. Isomerase
C. Aromatase D. Hydroxylase

169. Which of the following statements can be regarded as primary action of inhibin ?

A. It inhibits secretion of prolactin
B. It stimualtes synthesis of estradiol
C. It stimulates secretion of TSH
D. It inhibits secretion of FSH

170. Osteoclasts are inhibited by :

A. Parathyroid hormone
B. Calcitonin
C. 1, 25-dihydroxycholecalciferol
D. Tumor necrosis factor

171. All of the following hormones have cell surface reeptors except :

A. Adrenaline B. Growth Hormone
C. Insulin D. Thyroxine

172. Oral hypoglycemic with short half life is :

A. Glipizide B. Chlorpropamide
C. Acetohexamide D. Metformin

173. Which one of the following oral hypoglycemic agents has the longest duration of action :

A. Tolazamide B. Tolbutamide
C. Phenformin D. Chlorpropamide

174. Long term steroid treatment results in :

A. Resorption of bone matrix
B. Decreased vitamin D activation
C. Decreased Calcium loss of Urine
D. Increased calcium absorption from gut

175. Drug which increase the activity of oral contraceptives is :

A. Ethambutol B. Sulphonamide
C. Pyrazinamide D. Streptomycin

Ans.	167. C	168. C	169. D	170. B	171. D	172. D
	173. D	174. A	175. B			

176. The effect of oral contraceptive is decreased by all except :

A. Phenytoin B. Phenobarbitone
C. Rifampicin D. Chloropheniramine

177. All of the following statements regarding insulin resistance are true except :

A. Resistance develops on intermittent treatment with insulin
B. Seen in acromegaly
C. Seen in pheochromocytoma
D. Commoner with use of Humilin insulin (of bacterial origin)

178. One of the following insulin has longest duration of action :

A. Isophane insulin
B. Ultra lente (insulin zinc suspension)
C. Plain insulin
D. Lente insulin

179. Synthetic thyroid releasing hormone stimualtes release of all but one of the following :

A. Prolactin B. Follicular stimulating hormone
C. Growth hormone D. Adrenotrophin

180. One of the following sulfonylurea has active metabolite :

A. Tolbutamide B. Acetohexamide
C. Glibenclamide D. Glipizide

181. All of the following agents are used locally for spermicidal activity except

A. Phenylmercuric nitrate B. Chlorindanol
C. Danazol D. Hexylresorcinol

182. All except one increase the release of growth hormone :

A. Beta blocking drugs B. Alpha receptor blocking drugs
C. Vasopressin D. Estrogens

183. All except one are the uses of biguanides :

A. Indicated in maturity onset diabetes
B. In severe diabetics
C. In non-diabetic obese patients
D. In brittle juvenile diabetics

184. The steroid having the greatest anti-inflammatory potency

A. Hydrocortisone B. Prednisone
C. Dexamethasone D. Triamcinolone

185. Insulin accelerates glucose transport across mem- brane in :

A. Brain tissue B. Hepatic tissue
C. Intestinal muscle D. Erythrocytes

Ans.	176. D	177. A	178. B	179. D	180. B	181. C
	182. B	183. D	184. B	185. B		

186. Which of the following has the greatest rapidity of action ?

A. Thyroid extract
B. Sodium levothyroxine
C. Thyroxine
D. Trilodothyronine

187. Which of the following hormone does not need a second messenger :

A. Oestrogen
B. LH
C. FSH
D. Glucagon

188. Which of the following is orally effective :

A. Thyroxine
B. TSH
C. FSH
D. Insulin

189. Mechanism of action of propylthiouracil is to :

A. Inhibit iodine trapping
B. Inhibit tyrosine reuptake
C. Inhibit coupling of iodotyrosines
D. Inhibit metabolic resonse to T3

190. Which of the following drug is contraindicated in pheochromocytoma :

A. Guenethidine
B. Phenoxybenzamine
C. Labetelol
D. Propranolol

191. Immunosuppressive effect of cortisone is attributed to its ability to

A. Produce lymphopenia
B. Destroy immunoglobulin
C. Block DNA synthesis
D. Crosslink DNA strand

192. The drug of choice of treatment of diabetes insipidus is :

A. Desmopressin
B. Diazoxide
C. Thiazide diuretics
D. Chlorpropamide

193. Mifepristone is used for :

A. Termination of pregnancy
B. Suppression of Lactation
C. Treatment of prostatic cancer
D. Treatment of post partum haemorrhage

194. Estrogen acts on :

A. Cell membrane
B. Nucleus
C. Mitochandria
D. Cytoplasmic receptor

195. Methiazole differs from propylthiouracil in that :

A. It is less protein bound
B. Less excreted in breast milk
C. Lower volume of distribution
D. Loss frequent dosage schedule

196. Antithyroid action of lugol's iodine is by inhibition of :

A. Iodide uptake
B. Peroxidase
C. Cytosine coupling
D. D-iodinase

Ans.	186. D	187. A	188. A	189. C	190. A	191. A
	192. A	193. A	194. B	195. D	196. A	

197. **Least antigenic type of insulin is :**
A. Isophane B. Lente
C. Humlin D. PZI

198. **Administration of suplhonamide may intensify the action of tolbutamide, through :**
A. Activation of the islets of pancreas
B. Direct action on the utilization of glucose
C. Synergistic action
D. Competing with tolbutamide in plasma protein binding

199. **Which of the following is not an adverse effect of cortisone therapy :**
A. Peptic ulceration B. Psychoses
C. Osteoporesis D. Hypoglycemia

200. **Which of the following drugs can produce Galactorrhoea by interfering with neuronal transmission in brain :**
A. Physiostigmine B. Levodopa
C. Chlordiazepoxide D. Chlorpromazine

201. **The only insulin preparation which can be given intravenously is :**
A. Isophane insulin B. Crystalline zinc insulin
C. Protamine zinc insulin D. Plain insulin

202. **Which of the following vitamins resemble hormone :**
A. Vitamin K B. Vitamin D
C. Vitamin A D. Vitamin E

203. **All of following precautions should be taken before prescribing glucocorticoids except :**
A. History of peptic ulceration B. History of allergy
C. History of diabetes D. History of hypertension

204. **In thyroid crisis all are given except :**
A. Iodine B. Iodides
C. Neomercazole D. Propranolol

205. **In a lady taking oral contraceptives, drug to be used to supress lactation is :**
A. Bromocriptine B. Clomiphene
C. High dose of oral pills D. None of the above

206. **Oral hypoglycemic agents :**
A. Have potent diuretic action, in addition to their plasma glucose-lowering action
B. Are indicated for use in insulin-dependent diabetic patient, to increase the response to injected insulin
C. Stimulate insulin secretion and increase the sensitivity of cell to insulin
D. Can be used during pregnancy for ketotoic patient that have shown a response to the glucose lowering action of these drugs

Ans.	197. C	198. D	199. D	200. D	201. D	202. B
	203. B	204. C	205. A	206. C		

207. Adrogens such as testosterone tend to :

A. Produces hypocalcemia
B. Increase protein synthesis
C. Suppress growth of prostatic carcinoma
D. Decrease electrolyte retention

208. The following is an oral hypoglycemic agents except :

A. Tolbutamide B. Dichlorophen
C. Chlorpropamide D. Phenformin

209. Corticosteroid aggravates all except :

A. Congenital adrenal hyperplasia
B. Hypertension
C. Peptic ulcer
D. Diabetes mellitus

210. Drugs helping in inducing ovulation are all except :

A. Tomoxifen B. Gonadotrophin
C. Clomiphene D. Progesterone

211. Contraindications of Adrenal steroids are all except :

A. Cushing's syndrome B. Marked osteoporosis
C. Severe hypertension D. Pituitary insufficiency

212. If diethylstillboestrol is given to a pregnant female, it causes :

A. Precocious puberty B. Premature closure of epiphysis
C. Jaundice D. Hirsutism

213. Oestrogen have to be avoided in lactating women because it :

A. Suppresses lactation
B. Crosses placenta and cause feminization
C. Causes cogenital abnormalities
D. Causes jaundice

214. Following drug may cause Lactic acidosis :

A. Biguanides B. Glibenclamide
C. Tolbutamide D. Chlorpropamide

215. Therepeutic indication of oral contraceptive is all except :

A. Suppression of lactation B. Atrophic rhinitis
C. Fibrocystic disease of breast D. Stein Leventhal syndrome

216. Longest acting insulin is :

A. Protamine B. Benzathine
C. Crytalline D. None

217. Drug which causes hypothyroidism :

A. Lithium B. Carbamazepine
C. Methotrexate D. Sulphur

Ans.	**207. B**	**208. B**	**209. A**	**210. D**	**211. D**	**212. B**
	213. A	**214. A**	**215. D**	**216. A**	**217. A**	

218. **The preferred drug for confirming the presence of pheochromocytoma in a patient who is severely hypertensive is :**
A. Piperoxan B. Phenoxybenzamine
C. Histamine D. Phentolamine

219. **Highly purified insulin is used in the following conditions except :**
A. Diabetic nephropathy B. Insulin allergy
C. Insulin resistance D. Insulin lipodystrophy

220. **2nd generation sulfonylurea is :**
A. Tolbutamide B. Glibenclamide
C. Chlorpropamide D. Metformin

221. **Drug having structure like steroid is :**
A. ACTH B. Insulin
C. Chloromycetin D. Cyproterone

222. **Anti-inflammatory action of corticosteroid is directly proportional to :**
A. Glucocorticoid activity B. Mineralocorticoid activity
C. Both D. None of the above

223. **Treatment of choice of de Querian thyroiditis :**
A. Antithyroid drugs B. Propranolol
C. Thyroxine D. Prednisolone

224. **Management of acute hypercalcemia can be achieved with :**
A. Saline-infusion alone
B. Saline infusion with loop agents of EDTA
C. Administration of parathormone
D. Administration of calcitonin
E. Vit. D

225. **Drug which increases the activity of oral contraceptives is :**
A. Rifamicin B. Benzthiazide
C. Pyrazinamide D. Streptomycin

226. **One of the following progestational preparation has estrogenic effect also :**
A. Dehydrogesterone B. Medroxyprogesterone acetate
C. Ethynodiol D. Norethynodiol

227. **High levels of growth hormone are found in all but one of the following :**
A. Acromegaly B. Malnutritioned children
C. Myxoedema D. In prediabetic state

228. **Pharmacotherapy of an ovulatory infertility involves the use of :**
A. Ergonovine B. Bromocriptine
C. Clomiphene citrate D. Oxytocin

Ans.	218. D	219. A	220. B	221. D	222. A	223. D
	224. B	225. A	226. D	227. C	228. C	

E. PG FX

229. All of the following have mineralocorticoid effect except :

A. Hydrocortisone
B. Cortisone
C. Fluprodnislone
D. Prednisolone

230. One of the following inhibits action of androgen at the target tissue level :

A. Aminoglutethimide
B. Metypirone
C. Cyproterone acetate
D. Oxymetholone

231. Following hormones are increased in response to trauma and stress except :

A. Insulin
B. Cortisol
C. Adrenaline
D. GH

232. All of the following drugs inhibit release of insulin except :

A. Thaizides
B. Sulphonylureas
C. Diphenylhydantoin
D. Diazoxide

233. Currently used antithyroid drugs include the following except :

A. Methimazole
B. Potassium perchlorate
C. Carbimzole
D. Propylthiouracil

234. The drug of choice for Addison's disease is :

A. Hydrocortisone
B. Betamethasone
C. Dexamethasone
D. Prednisolone

235. All of the following are adverse effects of prolonged administration of high doses of thyroid hormone except :

A. Heat intoleranc
B. Exophthalmos
C. Palpitations
D. Lethargy

236. Somatostatin inhibits all except :

A. Insulin
B. GH
C. Thyroxine
D. Epinephrine

237. Corticosteroids act by :

A. Preventing membrane phospholipase activity
B. Inhibits thromboxane
C. Cyclooxygenase inhibitor
D. Prevent degranulation

238. Estrogen treatment is associated with :

A. Hepatocellular carcinoma
B. Hepatocellular adenoma
C. Bile duct adenoma
D. Cholangiocarcinoma

239. All of the following drugs produce galactorrhoea except :

A. Chlorpromazine
B. Thioridazine
C. Bromocriptine
D. Haloperidol

Ans.	229. C	230. C	231. A	232. B	233. B	234. A
	235. B	236. D	237. A	238. B	239. C	

240. Oral contraceptives do not increase hepatic meta-bolism of which drug

A. Rifampicin
B. Corticosteroids
C. Digoxin
D. Warfarin

241. The side effect of clomiphene is :

A. Fibroadenosis
B. Multiple pregnancy
C. Dysmenorrhoea
D. Dyspareunia

242. The half life of intravenous plain insulin is :

A. 15-30 sec.
B. 1—3 minutes
C. 5—7 minutes
D. 15—30 minutes

243. Hypoglycemia may be caused by :

A. Alcohol
B. Diazoxide
C. Thiazide
D. CPZ

244. All of the following statements about Human insulin are true except :

A. More effective in preventing complications of diabetes than animal insulins
B. Safer is patients who are allergic to animal insulin
C. Faster absorption and quicker action
D. Produced by recombinant DNA techniques

245. Human insulin differs from beef insulin by —— amino acids :

A. 1
B. 2
C. 3
D. 10

246. True about carbimazole (thiouracil) is :

A. It prevents I_2 binding
B. Acts immediately
C. Causes agranulocytosis
D. Rapidly absorbed

247. Hypoglycemia is least likely with :

A. Biguanides
B. Chlorpropamide
C. Glibenclamide
D. Tolbutamide

248. Antithyroid drug may be given in pregnant female :

A. Carbimazole
B. Methimazole
C. Propylthiouracil
D. Radioactive iodine

249. The first hormone, which is raised after injury is :

A. Thyroxine
B. Catecholamine
C. Growth hormone
D. LH

250. Glucose absorption is blocked by :

A. Quabain
B. Buformin
C. Tolbutamide
D. Diazoxide

251. Insulin acts through receptors :

A. β1 adrenergic
B. β2 adrenergic
C. α and β
D. α only

Ans.	240. C	241. B	242. C	243. A	244. A	245. C
	246. C	247. D	248. C	249. B	250. B	251. C

252. All of the following are the side effects of tHMG + HCG except :

A. Ascites B. Intraperitoneal bleeding

C. Vaginal bleeding D. Electrolyte imbalance

253. The principle afferent receptors for the neural control of ACTH in response to hypovolemia lie in :

A. Skin B. Muscles

C. Peripheral blood vessels D. Right atrium

254. One of the following does not have diurnal variation in its blood levels :

A. Growth hormone

B. ACTH (Adrenocorticotrophic hormone)

C. Thyroid stimulating hormone

D. Prolactin

255. Drugs used for medical castration is :

A. FSH B. FSH antagonist

C. LHRH agonist D. Aminogluthemide

256. The effects of hypoglycemia is masked by :

A. Heparin

B. Cephalosporins

C. Calcium channel blockers

D. None of the above

257. Chlopropamide metabolism is enthanced by :

A. Ethyl alcohol B. Diazepam

C. Lorazepam D. Chlordiazepoxide

258. Dexamethasone is — times potent than cortisone :

A. 3 B. 10

C. 30 D. 50

259. Human pituitary gonadotropins differ from human chorionic gonadotropins in one of the following ways :

A. Can cause ovulation

B. Can stimualte follicular growth

C. Maintain pregnancy

D. Ineffective in primary ovarion failure

260. Endocrine manifestations as a side effect are caused by :

A. Fluconazole B. Ketoconazole

C. Itraconazole D. Thiabendazol

261. Most common side effect of prolonged use of steroids is :

A. Affective disorders B. Confusion

C. Delirium D. Schizophrenia

Ans.	252. D	253. D	254. C	255. C	256. D	257. A
	258. C	259. B	260. B	261. A		

262. **Clinical applications of ACTH includes :**
A. Treatment of Addison's disease
B. Diagnostic agent
C. Reduction of adrenal ascorbie acid
D. Treatment of Ketosis

263. **Following are the actions of diazoxide except :**
A. Stimulates release of catecholamines
B. Stimulates release of insulin
C. Increase glucose uptake by the liver ·
D. Causes water retention

264. **Which drugs are effective in the absence of a functioning adrenal gland?**
A. Cortisone B. Dexamethasone
C. Both D. Neither

265. **Which of the following best describes the action of desoxycorticosterone (DOC) ?**
A. Is a potent antiinflammatory agent
B. Promotes K+ reabsorption in the distal renal tuble
C. Has no effect on water or electolyte excretion
D. Promotes Na+ reabsorption in the distal tubule

266. **All of the following acts on protein regulation through nuclear receptor except :**
A. GnRH B. Estrogen
C. Androgen D. Progesteron

267. **Major site of action of insulin are all except :**
A. Muscle B. Adipose tissue
C. Liver D. Kidney

268. **The primary mechanism of ACTH is :**
A. Stimulation of CRF release
B. Stimulation of steroidogenesis
C. Release of stored cortisol
D. Antagonism of aldosterone activity

269. **The abuse of anabolic steroids by male athletes can result in all of the following except :**
A. Anorexia B. Decreased spermatogenesis
C. Ferminization D. Retention of fluid

270. **Chemical structure of chorionic gonadotropic is common to all but one of the following :**
A. LH (Leutenising hormone)
B. FSH (Follicular stimulating hormone)
C. TSH (Thyroid stimulating hormone)
D. Oxytocin

Ans.	262. B	263. B	264. C	265. D	266. A	267. D
	268. B	269. C	270. D			

271. Dose of levo-thyroxine is :
A. 100 mg B. 10 mg
C. 1 mg D. 0.1 mg

272. c-GMP is second messenger for :
A. Insulin B. Thyroxine
C. GH D. FSH

273. DOC is Ca Thyroid :
A. Methotrexate B. Vincritine
C. 5-FU D. Doxorubicin

274. Mode of action of steroidal contraceptive is :
A. ↑ LH B. ↓ LH
C. ↑ FSH D. ↑ LH & FSH

275. Insulin from human preferred because :
A. Allergic reactions less B. Hypoglycemia infrequent
C. Longer acting D. Edema less common

276. Steroid with only glucocorticoid activity is :
A. Fludrocortisone B. Triamcilone
C. Prednisolone D. Hydrocortisone

277. Calcitonin is given in following except :
A. Renal osteodysplasia B. Hyperparathyroidism
C. Hyper vitamenosis D D. Paget's disease

278. Tamoxifen is maximum useful in :
A. Estrogen `+' ve Ca breast B. Ca lung
C. Ca liver D. Testicular Ca

279. Wrong about bromocriptine is :
A. Dopamine agonist B. ↑ Prolactin secretion
C. Causes nausea & vomiting D. All of the above

280. Glucagon receptors are on :
A. Cell membrane B. Cytoplasm
C. Nucleus D. Cell wall

281. Syndrome of inappropiate ADH secretion (SIADH) is caused by :
A. Acetohexamide B. Chlorpropamide
C. Tolbutamide D. Glipizide

282. Prolonged steroid therapy causes following except :
A. ↓ incidence of infection
B. Suppression of pituitary adrenal axis
C. Psychosis
D. ↓ muscle mass

283. Insulinoma is diagnosed by :
A. Phenformin B. Insulin
C. Tolbutamide D. Glucagon

Ans.	271. D	272. A	273. D	274. B	275. A	276. B
	277. A	278. A	279. B	280. A	281. B	282. D
	283. C					

284. Anabolic steroids may produce the following side effects except :

A. Precocious puberty in children
B. Cholestatic jaundice
C. Delayed closure of epiphysis in children
D. Acne in males and females

285. Hormones acting on cAMP as second messenger are following except :

A. MSH & HCG
B. NE & LH
C. PTH & TSH
D. Insulin & Thyroxin

286. Immunosuppressive effect of cortisone is attributed to its ability to :

A. Produce lymphopenia
B. Destroy immunoglobulin
C. Block DNA synthesis
D. Crosslink DNA strand

287. Which of the following is not an indication for starting sulfonylurea therapy:

A. Total pancreatectomy
B. Late onset of disease
C. Obesity
D. Duration of disease less than 5 years

288. Which is contraindicated in pheochromocytoma.

A. Prazosin
B. Atenolol
C. Nitropruside
D. Metyrosine

289. Not a progesterone is :

A. Mestronol
B. Megesterol
C. Dehydrogesterone
D. Norgesterol

290. About T3 & T4 true all except :

A. T4 is less potent than T3
B. T4 is better absorbed than T3
C. Conc. Of T4 more than T3
D. T4 binds to plasma protein more than T3

291. In diabetic coma, the drug of choice is :

A. Crystalline Insulin
B. Lente Insulin
C. Protamine Zinc Insulin
D. Ultra Lente Insulin

292. The following are ovulation inducing drugs except :

A. Bromo ergocriptine
B. Clomiphene citrate
C. Danazol
D. Cyclofenil

293. Corticosteroids are indicated in all except :

A. T.B. intestine
B. T.B. Meningitis
C. T.B. Kidney
D. T.B. Pleura

294. The corticosteroid preferred for use in Addison's disease is :

A. Aldosterone
B. Fludrocortisone
C. Hydrocortisone
D. Betamethasone

Ans.						
	284. C	**285. D**	**286. A**	**287. A**	**288. B**	**289. A**
	290. B	**291. A**	**292. C**	**293. A**	**294. B**	

295. Which of the following antidiabetic drugs inhibits intestinal brush border glucosidase enzymes ?

A. Acarbose
B. Troglitazone
C. Metformin
D. Guargum

296. Metabolic rate of which of the following organs is not significantly affected by thyroxine ?

A. Brain,
B. Heart
C. Liver
D. Skeletal muscle

297. Antagonists of adrenocoritcal agents include the following except :

A. Metyrapone
B. Metyrosine
C. Aminoglutelhimide
D. Mitotane
E. Amphenone B

298. The endocrine effects or insulin include the following except :

A. Inhibits glycogenolysis
B. Inhibits the conversion of fatty acids to keto acids
C. Inhibits conversion of amino acids to glucose
D. Decreases triglyceride synthesis and VLDL formation
E. Increases the synthesis of glycogen in the muscle

299. True of tamoxifen :

A. Binds to estrogen receptors
B. ↑ estrogen production
C. ↓ FSH prosduction
D. ↑ LH secretion

300. Which of the following is not an indication for oxytocin :

A. Premature labour
B. Post partum haemorrhage
C. Uterine inertia
D. Breast engorgement due to inefficient milk ejection reflex

301. True statement about thyroxine in circulation is :

A. T4 is mainly bound to the thyroxine binding globulin
B. Normal proportion of free T4 is 10 times greater than T3
C. T3 is strongly bound to the TBPA
D. Reverse T3 is synthesized in acini but is not released in circulation

302. Glucocorticoids causes all except :

A. Muscle wasting
B. Osteoporosis
C. Diabetes mellitus
D. Reduced appetite

303. Corticosteroid which need least systemic monitoring is :

A. Prednisolone
B. Budesonide
C. Hydrocortisone
D. Dexamethasone

Ans. **295. A** **296. A** **297. B** **298. D** **299. A** **300. A** **301. A** **302. D** **303. B**

304. **Drug used in diabetes is :**
A. Salmeterol
B. Acetohexamide
C. Benserazide
D. Methoxamin

W.305 **Drug producing SIADH is :**
A. Carbimazepine
B. Cisplatin
C. Cyclophosphamide
D. Methotrexate

306. **All the following are true of the use of oral hypogly-cemic agents except :**
A. Ethanol blunts the action of sulfonyureas
B. Long acting sulfonyurea causes hypoglycemia
C. Metformin is contraindicated in renal failure
D. Thiazolidonediones acts by decreasing insulin resistance & increasing glucose utilization

307. **Steroids are not indicated in the treatment of :**
A. Hypercalcemia
B. Respiratory distress
C. Intraventricular haemorrhage
D. Enterocolitis

308. **All are true about Metformin except :**
A. Causes lactic acidosis both indiabetic and non-diabetic
B. Acts by increased insulin secretion
C. Increases peripheral utilisation of glucose and decreases absorption of glucose
D. When given with diethyl alcohol, increased risk of lactic acidemia.

309. **The following drugs cause hypertensive crisis in phaeochromocytoma except :**
A. Phenoxybenzamine
B. Propranolol
C. Saralasin
D. Captopril

310. **All are true about statins except :**
A. Fluvastatin and simvastatin are redistributed to CNS
B. Pravastatin rapidly metabolised
C. Fluvastatin and simvastatin are longer acting than Pravastatin
D. Lovastatin and simvastatin are hydrophilic.

311. **Steroids cause the following except :**
A. Hypertrophy of muscles
B. Hypokalemia
C. Neuropsychiatirc
D. Hyperglycemia

312. **Tamoxifen used in the treatment of breast carcinoma leads to :**
A. Osteoporosis
B. Endometrial hyperplasia
C. Fibroadenoma breast
D. Ovarian tumours

313. **All the following complications are seen with use of oral contraceptives except :**
A. MI
B. Venous thrombosis
C. Stroke
D. Intracranial hemorrhage

Ans.	304. B	305. A,B	306. A	307. A	308. A	309. A
	310. B	311. A	312. B	313. D		

314. Insulin mediated glucose entry is most important in which of the following organs :

A. Erythrocytes
B. Hepatocytes
C. Brain
D. Muscle

315. Corticosteroids given to mother prevent all the following complications in the newborn except :

A. Hyaline membrane disease
B. Intraventricular hemorrhage
C. Necrotizing enterocolitis
D. Bronchopulmonary aplasia

316. Which of the following act via cAMP :

A. LH
B. Testosterone
C. Thyroxin
D. Estrogen

317. Epinephrine causes glycogenolysis by :

A. Adenyl cyclase
B. Conversion of diphospoglycogen synthase to phosphoglycogen synthase
C. Phosphorylase
D. Adenyl kinase

318. All the following belong to the steroid receptor superfamily except :

A. Vitamin D3 receptor
B. Thyroid receptor
C. Retinoid receptor
D. Epinephrine receptor

319. The following hormone does not have any intracellular receptor :

A. Vitamin D2
B. Cortisone
C. Adrenaline
D. Thyroxine

320. Bovine insulin can causes all except :

A. Lipodystrophy
B. Obesity
C. Hyperpigmentation
D. Allergy

321. All of the following statements about an alpha-glucosidase inhibitor are true except?

A. Reduces intestinal absorption of carbohydrates
B. Effective in both type 1 and type 2 diabetes mellitus
C. Hypoglycemia is a common and serious side effect
D. Can be used with other oral hypoglycemic agents

322. Which one of the following statements about biguanides is not true?

A. Do not stimulate insulin release
B. Decrease hepatic glucose production
C. Renal dysfunction is not a contraindication for their use
D. Can be combined with sulfonylureas

Ans.	**314. D**	**315. D**	**316. A**	**317. A**	**318. D**	**319. C**
	320. B	**321. C**	**322. C**			

323. **All of the following appear to decrease hot flushes in menopausal women except :**

A. Androgens
B. Raloxifene
C. Isoflavaones
D. Tibolone

324. **A 46 year old male patient has cushing's Syndrome that is due to the presence of following drugs would be expected to reduce the signs and symptoms of this man' di :**

A. Betamethasone B. Cortisol
C. Fludrocortisol D. Ketoconozole

325. **Weight of normal adult adrenal gland is about ——— gm :**

A. 2 B. 5
C. 7 D. 12

326. **Pseudohypoparathyroidism is characterised by the following except :**

A. Hypocalcemia
B. Hyperphosphatemia
C. Response to injected parathyroid hormone
D. Developmental abnormallities

327. **Thyroid hormones release into circulation occurs due to :**

A. Phagocytosis
B. Osmosis of hormones
C. Lysosomal digestion of colloid droplets
D. Enzymatic chain reaction

328. **Thyroglossal cyst arise in neck in :**

A. Anterior midline
B. Right lateral midline
C. Left lateral midline
D. Any where

329. **Thyroglossal cyst may occasionally give rise to ——— carcinoma :**

A. Papillary B. Medullary
C. Anaplastic D. Follicular

330. **Aldactone therapy rsults in eosinophilic cyloplasmic bodies (2-20m) in**

A. Zona glomerulosa B. Zona reticulata
C. Zona fasciculata D. Adrenal medulla

331. **Spironolactone bodies are altered :**

A. Lysosomes B. Nucleolus
C. Mitochondria D. Lysosomes

Ans.	323. B	324. D	325. B	326. C	327. C	328. A
	329. A	330. A	331. C			

332. Most frequent site of spread of adrenal cortical carcinomas is :

A. Liver B. Lungs
C. Lymph nodes D. Bone

333. Commonest presentation of Endemic goitre :

A. Asymptomatic B. Hypothyroidism
C. Lump in neck D. Hyperthyroidism

334. Cushings syndrome is most commonly seen in :

A. Bronchogenic Carcinoma B. Renal Cell Carcinoma
C. Pancreatic Carcinoma D. Lymphoma

335. The levels of 17-ketosteroids in urine is increased in :

A. Adrenal tumour only
B. Adrenal and Testicular tumour
C. Liver Secondaries
D. Bronochogenic carcinoma

336. Commonest cause of ambiguous genitalia is :

A. Klinefelters syndrome B. 21-hydroxylase deficiency
C. Mixed gonadal dysgenesis D. Testicular feminisation

337. Tumour marker for Endodermal sinus tumour :

A. CEA B. HCG
C. Alpha feto protein D. Cytokeratin

338. Most common islet cell tumour :

A. Insulinoma B. Gastrinoma
C. Glucagonoma D. Somatostatinoma

339. Pituitary adenomas show the following histological pattern except :

A. Papillary B. Diffuse
C. Adenoid cystic D. Sinusoidal

340. In Phaeochromocytoma, excretion of which of the following is increased ?

A. Urinary VMA B. Serum bradykinin
C. Plasma HMA D. All of the above

341. Massive Adrenal metastasis is most common in which of the following lung tumor :

A. Squamous cell tumor B. Oat cell tumor
C. Bronchial adenoma D. Undifferentiated carcinoma

342. Weight range of adrenal glands in most of the cases of Cushing's disease is :

A. 4-11 gm B. 11-13 gm
C. 14-24 gm D. 24-30 gm

Ans.	332. B	333. C	334. A	335. B	336. B	337. C
	338. A	339. D	340. A	341. D	342. D	

343. **Commonest pathological cause of hypercorticism is :**
A. Hyperplasia B. Adenoma
C. Carcinoma D. T.B.

344. **Cushing's syndrome may be seen in :**
A. Oat cell carcinoma of lung
B. Thymomas
C. Medullary thyroid carcinoma
D. Islet cell carcinoma
E. Any of the above

345. **Commonest cause of primary adrenal insufficiency in India is :**
A. Addison's disease B. Congenital
C. Iatrogenic D. T.B.

346. **Renal lesions in hyperparathyroidism are the following except :**
A. Nephrocalcinosis B. Renal stones
C. Amyloidosis D. Pyelonephritis

347. **Most frequent extra-adrenal site of pheochro-mocytoma is :**
A. Retroperitoneum (Organs of Zuckerkandle)
B. Post. mediastinum
C. Anal region
D. Urinary bladder

348. **Normal thyroid weight varies —— with dietary iodine content :**
A. Directly proportional B. Inversely
C. Inverse cubically D. Not fixed

349. **Average weight of thyroid gland where diet is rich in iodine is :**
A. 10-12 gm B. 14-16 gm
C. 18-20 gm D. 28-30 gm

350. **In Hashimoto's thyroiditis, infiltrate is predominantly :**
A. Eosinophilic B. Basophitic
C. Lymphocytic D. Neutrophilic

351. **In Hashimoto's disease, serum antibodies are mainly against :**
A. Thyroid follicles B. Thyrodine
C. Thyroglobulins D. Iodine

352. **Riedel's struma is histologically characterized by all except :**
A. Granulomatous inflammation
B. Lymphocytes and plasma cells
C. Thyroid is locally replaced by fibrous tissue
D. Sclerosis of blood vessels

353. **In papillary carcinoma, iodine intake is —— as compared to normal thyroid tissue :**
A. Increased
B. Reduced

Ans.	343. A	344. E	345. D	346. C	347. A	348. B
	349. C	350. C	351. C	352. A	353. B	

C. Reduced followed by increased
D. No change

354. Increased glycogen in chief cells of uninvolved parathyroid is seen in :
A. Parathyroid chief cell adenoma
B. Pri. chief cell hyperplasia
C. Multiple adenoma
D. Milk alkali syndrome of Burnett

355. Hypoparathyroidism is sometimes associated with hypofunction of :
A. Adrenal cortex B. Adrenal medulla
C. Thyroid D. Pancreas

356. Which of the following is most often involved in Multiple Endocrine Neoplasia I :
A. Pituitary B. Pancreas
C. Parathyroid D. Thyroid

357. Differential diagnosis of Solitary nodule thyroid includes following except :
A. Follicular carcinoma B. Adenoma
C. Anaplastic carcinoma D. Cyst

358. Histopathological indicator of malignancy in phaeochromocytoma ?
A. Increased mitotic activity B. Pleomorphism
C. Vascular invasion D. High nuclear index

359. Commonest cause of primary hyperparathyroidism :
A. Adenoma B. Carcinoma
C. Hyperplasia D. Renal failure

360. Which of the following histologic types of thyroid carcinoma carries the best prognosis ?
A. Follicular carcinoma B. Papillary carcinoma
C. Medullary carcinoma D. Malignant lymphoma

361. This non-endocrine tumor is known to secrete hormones :
A. Oat cell carcinoma of the lung
B. Rhabdomysarcoma of uterus
C. Carcinoma of the stomach
D. Adenomatoid tumor of the testis

362. Autoimmune thyroid disorders are usually associated with :
A. Hypothyroidism
B. Antithyroglobulin antibodies
C. Antimicrosomal antibodies
D. All of the above

Ans.	354. A	355. A	356. C	357. C	358. C	359. A
	360. B	361. A	362. D			

363. **Most common type of thyroid carcinoma is :**
A. Papillary B. Fomcular
C. Medullary D. Anaplastic

364. **The function of acini in thyroid is synthesis of :**
A. Tyrosine B. Thyroxine
C. Thyroglobuin D. Mucus

365. **Bronze Diabetes (consisting of pigmentary liver tint of skin) is seen in :**
A. Niemann pick disease B. Gaucher's disease
C. Haemochromatosis D. CCl4 intoxication
E. Chronic lead poisoning

366. **Medullary carcinoma thyroid is associated with :**
A. Amyloid stroma B. Based cell carcinoma
C. Calcitonin D. A+C

367. **Hurthle cells are seen in :**
A. Hashimoto's thyroiditis B. Granulomatous thyroiditis
C. Riedel's struma D. Acute thyroditis

368. **All are true of de Queruain's thyroiditis except :**
A. Increased ESR B. Increased I^{131} uptake
C. Pain D. Fever

369. **APUD cells are present in :**
A. Bronchus B. Pancreas
C. Appendix D. All of the above

370. **From which of the following does pheochromocytoma not arise :**
A. Adrenal medulla B. Adrenal cortex
C. Extra adrenal sites D. Sympahtetic chain

371. **Tumour which has most extensive endocrine paraneoplastic effects :**
A. Oat cell carcinoma B. Squamous cell
C. Large cell D. Adenocarcinoma

W.372. **Tumors that may produce substances with the hormone activity include :**
A. Oat cell carcinoma of the bronchus
B. Medullary carcinoma thyroid
C. Granulosa-theca cell tumor of the ovary
D. Renal cell carcinoma

W.373. **Adrenal cortex in the adreno-genital syndrome shows :**
A. Hyperplasia mainly of zona fasiculata
B. Hyperplasia of Zona reticularis
C. Hyperplasia mainly Zona glomerulosa
D. Adrenal cortical atrophy

Ans.	363. A	364. C	365. C	366. D	367. A	368. B
	369. D	370. B	371. A	372. ALL	373. A,D	

374. A small thyroid gland is seen in all of the following except :

A. Individuals over 50 years of age
B. Congenital cretinism
C. Granulomatous thyroiditis
D. Riedel's struma

375. All are true regarding carcinoid syndrome except :

A. Common site is appendix
B. Involve whole of the GIT except rectum
C. Flushing is common symptom
D. Secreted neurohormones

376. All are seen in Turner's Syndrome except :

A. Mental Retardation
B. Short stature
C. Infertility
D. Coarctation of Aorta

377. All of the following secrete hormones except :

A. Teratoma
B. Choriocarcinoma
C. Seminoma
D. Dysgerminoma

378. Which of the following chromosomal pattern is characteristic of testicular feminizing syndrome :

A. 48 XX
B. 48 XY
C. 47 XXY
D. 46 XY

379. True about papillary carcinoma of thyroid :

A. Encapsulated
B. Amyloid seen
C. Vacuolations in nucleus
D. 10-15 percent of thyroid malignancies

380. A middle aged female with increased T3, T4 & TSH. all are consistent findings with following except :

A. Diffuse goitre
B. Hashimoto's thyroiditis
C. Reidel's struma
D. MNG

381. Parathyroid hyperplasia is differentiated from parathyroid adenoma by :

A. Chief cells predominate
B. During surgery, all four glands are hyperplastic
C. Vascular invasion
D. Electron microscopy

382. Best screeening test for hyperthyroidism :

A. Serum TRH& TSH estimatin
B. Serum TSH .T4 estimatn
C. Radioactive iodine uptake
D. Serum T3. T4

Ans.	374. C	375. B	376. A	377. C	378. C	379. C
	380. C	381. A	382. D			

383. Type I diabetus mellitus is associated with all the following except :

A. Insulitis
B. Reduction in B cell mass
C. B cell degranulation
D. Amyloid change in B cells

384. Which of the following gene defects is associated with development of Medullary carcinoma of Thyroid?

A. Ret proto Oncogene
B. FAP gene
C. Rb gene
D. BRCA 1 gene

385. The most common histologic type of Thyroid cancer is?

A. Medullary type
B. Follicular type
C. Papillary type
D. Anaplastic type

386. Which one of the following investigations is most sensitive for early diagnosis of diabetic-nephropathy ?

A. Serum creatinine level
B. Creatinine clearance
C. Glucose Tolerance Test
D. Microalbuminuria

387. Gynaecomastia may be observed in patients with except :

A. Digitalis therapy
B. Klinefelter's syndrome
C. Aldacotone therapy
D. Cirrhosis of the liver
E. None of the above

388. Thiocyanates and perchlorates interfere with :

A. Iodination of tyrosine
B. Release of thyroxine
C. Release of tri-iodothyronine
D. Trapping of iodine by thyroid

389. Adrenogenital syndrome (congenital adrenal hyperplasia) may be produced by the deficiency of the following enzymes except :

A. C-21 hydroxylase
B. C-11 hydroxylase
C. 3-Beta hydroxydehydrogenase
D. C-18 dehydrogenase
E. Aldolase

390. In the treatment of thyrotoxic crisis all the drugs mentioned may be used except :

A. Hydrocortisone
B. Propranolol
C. Iodine
D. Chlorpromazine
E. Salbutamol

391. The usual number of parathyroid gland is :

A. One
B. Two
C. Four
D. Six
E. Eight

Ans.	383. C	384. A	385. C	386. D	387.E	388.D
	389.E	390.E	391.C			

392. True about Calcitonin is all except :

A. In normal humans is produced exclusively by the para follicular cells of the thyroid
B. Reduces the number and activity of osteoclasts
C. Reduces renal tubular reabsorption of calcium
D. Reduced renal tubular reabsorption of phosphate
E. If present in excess commonly causes tetany

393. In Cushing's syndrome false is :

A. Muscular wasting affects proximal muscles more than distal ones
B. More than half the patients are hypertensive at the time of diagnosis
C. Eosinophilia is common
D. Hypokalaemia is suggestive of a malignant cause
E. If a pituitary microadenoma is the cause its removal may be expected to restore normal ACTH function

394. Secondary hyperparathyroidism is seen with :

A. CRF B. Single adenoma
C. Metastasis in bone D. Potassium sparing diuretics

95. Hypoglycaemic effect of soluble insulin lasts for :

A. 12-20 hours B. 20-30 hours
C. 0.5 - 1.0 hour D. 6-10 hours
E. 2-4 hours

96. Maximum hyperprolactinemia is een in :

A. Bromocriptine therapy B. Chlorpromazine therapy
C. Reseripine therapy D. Pituitary adenoma

97. Which of the following is not associated with tetany ?

A. Chovostek's sign B. Trousseau's sign
C. Erb's sign D. Coles's sign
E. Personeal sign

98. Hyperaldosteronism causes :

A. Hyperkalemia B. Hyponatremia
C. Decreased water absorption D. Hypokalemia

99. Keroacidosis without glycosuria is seen in :

A. Aspirin toxicity B. Renal tubular acidosis
C. Starvation of long duration D. Acute renal failure

400. Which of the following are not related to myxoedema ?

A. Coronary atherosclerosis
B. Type III hyperlipoproteinaemia
C. Pericardial effusion
D. Often cardiac temponade

Ans.	392.E	393.C	394.A	395.D	396.D	397.D
	398.D	399.C	400.D			

401. **Weight gain is seen in following except :**
A. Pheachromocytoma
B. Cushing syndrome
C. Hypothyroidism
D. Hypersecretion of insulin

402. **Hyperpigmentation and pituitary enlargement after bilateral adrenalectomy is :**
A. Sheehan's syndrome
B. Cushing syndrome
C. Nelson's syndrome
D. Frohlich syndrome

403. **A 35 years old lady presents with a B.P. of 140/96 mm Hg. Her systemic examination was normal . She has :**
A. Cushing syndrome
B. Conn' s syndrome
C. Phaeochromocytoma
D. None of the above

404. **Most common presentation of primary Hyperpara-thyroidism is :**
A. Gall stones
B. Subtle neurological and Psychiatric symptoms
C. Abdominal pain
D. Recurrent abortion

405. **In Non ketotic hyperosmolar hyperglycemia, the blood sugar level is :**
A. Slightly elevated
B. Mildy elevated
C. Moderately elevated
D. Grossly elevated

406. **Treatment of Hypercalcemia is following except :**
A. Riwzole
B. Plicamycin
C. Bisdionate
D. Gallium nitrate

407. **In Insulin resistance, associated is :**
A. Obesity
B. Antibodies for Insulin
C. Antibodies for Insulin receptor
D. All of the above

408. **Common cause of Cushing's syndrome :**
A. Pituitary adenoma
B. Ectopic ACTH production
C. Solitary parathyroid tumor
D. Bronchogenic Ca

409. **Common cause of hyperparathyroidism :**
A. Multiple parathyroid adenoma
B. Solitary parathyroid adenoma
C. Adrenal hyperplasia
D. Ectopic PTH production

410. **Follicular carcinoma-thyroid commonly metastasized through :**
A. Blood
B. Lymphatic
C. Synmonic
D. None of the above

Ans.	401.A	402.C	403.C	404.B	405.D	406.A
	407.D	408.A	409.B	410.A		

411. In the case of long standing multiple nodular thyroid, tumor which commonly develops :

A. Follicular CA
B. Adenolymphoma
C. Papillary CA
D. None of the above

412. Hyperpigmentation is not seen in :

A. Hypothyrodism
B. Hypoadrenalism
C. Cushing's disease
D. Graves disease

413. SIADH occur in :

A. Hypothyroidism
B. Hypogonadism
C. Hypopituitarism
D. Diabetes

W414. Following are seen in Primary thyrotoxicosis except :

A. Myopathy
B. Exophthalmos
C. Prebital myxedema
D. Diffuse goitre

415. Pendred syndrome refers to :

A. Endemic goitre + nerve deafness
B. Sporadic goitre + nerve deafness
C. Endemic goitre + conductive deafness
D. Sporadic goitre + conductive deafness

416. Diabetes insipidus is characterized by :

A. ↓ urine osmilality and ↑ plasma osmolality
B. ↑ urine osmolality and ↓ plasma osmolality
C. ↑ urine osmolality and ↑ plasma osmolality
D. ↓ urine osmolality and ↓ plasma osmolality

417. Azoospermia with raised FSH level is seen in :

A. Testicular failure
B. Hypothalamic failure
C. Obstruction of vas
D. Cryptorchidism

418. The resin T-3 uptake test may be raised in presence of all, except :

A. Anticoagulants
B. Androgens
C. Acidosis
D. Pregnancy

419. The treatment of choice for ambulatory patients with diabetes insipidus is :

A. Lysine vaspressin spray
B. Cholopropamide
C. Pitressin tannate in oil
D. Thiazides

420. Most common causes for the panhypopituitarism in the adult include all, except :

A. Craniopharyngioma
B. Chromophobe adenoma
C. Sarcoidosis
D. Postapartum pituitary necrosis and acromegaly (end stage)

Ans.	411.A	412.A	413.A	414.NONE	415.A	416.A
	417.A	418.D	419.A	420.C		

421. **Activity of acromegaly is suggested by all of the following except :**
A. Glucose intolerance
B. Lowered serum inorganic phosphorus
C. Raised basal levels of growth hormone
D. Increased excretion of hydroxyproline in urine

422. **All of the following increase growth hormone levels except :**
A. Vasopressin
B. Exercise
C. Hyperglycaemia
D. Prolonged fast

423. **Most sensitive assay for human growth hormone is :**
A. Mouse bioassay
B. Radioimmunoassay
C. Metapyrone test
D. Insulin tolerance test**ctors in**

424. **Factors in the pathogenesis of diabetic ketoacidosis include except :**
A. Raised growth hormone
B. Raised glucosteroids
C. Raised catecholamines
D. Raised insulin action

425. **Proinsulin can be best characterized as :**
A. Immunologically similar to insulin
B. Completely inactive
C. More active than insulin
D. Smaller than insulin

426. **In adrenal cortical hyperfunction all of the following may occur except :**
A. Hypertension
B. Hypernatremia
C. Diabetes mellitus
D. Sodium retention
E. Increased gluconeogenesis

427. **Consider the following cancers :**
1. Retroperitoneal fibrosarcoma
2. Carcinoid
3. Gastric carcinoma
4. Thyroid papillary carcinoma

Those associated with hypoglycemia due to the release of an insulin like substance would include :
A. 1 and 2
B. 3 and 4
C. 2 and 3
D. 1,2 and 4

428. **Characteristic feature of Cushing's syndrome include :**
A. Osteomalacia
B. Proximal muscle weakness
C. Menorrhagia
D. Hypotension
E. Generalized obesity

429. **True precocious puberty occurs in all except :**
A. Congenital adrenal Hyperplasia
B. Craniopharyngioma
C. Hypothalamic hamatoma
D. Albright syndrome

Ans.	421.B	422.C	423.B	424.D	425.A	426.A
	427.A	428.B	429.D			

430. Fibrocalculous pancreatic Diabetes is characterised by all of the following except :

A. History of Casawa consumption
B. Pancreatic calculi
C. Keto resistance
D. Low insulin requirement

431. Alcohol induced testicular atrophy :

A. Occurs often due to hepatic involvement
B. Occurs due to increase in blood viscosity
C. Occurs due to venoocclusion
D. Occurs secondary to peripheral neuropathy

432. Anti-diuretic hormone deficiency may result from :

A. Compulsive water drinking
B. Prolonged diuretic therapy
C. Eosinophilic granuloma
D. Multiple myeloma

433. Features of chronic thyroiditis includes all of the following, except :

A. Increased plasma gamma globulin
B. Weight gain
C. Circulating autoantibodies
D. Goitre
E. Low or normal PBI

434. The best test for distinguishing primary and secondary myxoedema is :

A. P.B.I B. B.E.I
C. TSH stimulation test D. B.M.R
E. Radioactive triiodothyronin resin uptake

435. With regard to precocious puberty :

A. Is never idiopathic
B. May be caused by thalamic tumours
C. It includes both menstruation and secondary sexual development before the age of 12
D. In males it is before 10 years and in females it is below 8 years

436. Absence of fructose in semen indicates :

A. Obstruction of Vas
B. Obstruction of ejaculatory duct
C. Testcular failure
D. Prostatic atrophy

Ans.	430.D	431.A	432.C	433.B	434.C	435.D
	436.B					

437. **All are true of the Quervain's thyroiditis except :**
A. Fever074
B. Local pain
C. Increased ESR
D. Increased radio iodine uptake

438. **IDDM is found to be associated with all the following except :**
A. Addison's disease B. SLE
C. Hashimoto's thyroiditis D. Muscular dystrophy

439. **Dysphagia with ptosis and generalized mucle weak-ness is seen in :**
A. Thyrotoxic myopathy
B. Muscular dystrophy
C. Myasthenia gravis
D. Hypokalemic periodic paralysis

440. **Following are true of Conn's syndrome except :**
A. Hypokalemia B. Low renin levels
C. Raised blood pressure D. Generalized edema

441. **The ocular muscle most commonly affected in Thyrotoxic myopathy is :**
A. Inferior rectus B. Inferior oblique
C. Superior rectus D. Superior oblique

442. **Acromegaly is characterized by all except :**
A. Enlarged nasal sinuses B. Increased heel pad thickness
C. Muscular hypertrophy D. Diabetes mellitus

443. **Blood sugar estimation is relevant in all of the following except :**
A. RH incompatibility B. Birth asphyxia
C. Large for date D. Baby of hypothyroid mother

444. **Neurological features associated with hypothyroidism include :**
A. Ataxia B. Carpal tunnel syndrome
C. Deafness D. All of the above

445. **Congenital 17 hydroxylase deficiency leads to :**
A. Virilism B. Hermaphroditism
C. Hypertension D. Hyperkalemia

446. **Highly purified insulin is used in the treatment of diabetics on a following instance except :**
A. Insulin allergy B. Diabetes nephropathy
C. Insulin lipodystrophy D. Insulin resistance

447. **Vasopressin deficiency leads to :**
A. Raised urinary osmolality
B. Hyponatremia
C. Decreased concentrating ability of kidney
D. Increased blood volume

Ans.	437.	438.D	439.C	440.D	441.D	442.C
	443.A	444.D	445.C	446.B	447.C	

448. Assertion—Diabetes insipidus, water loss may be > 20L/day Reason—ADH acts at proximal convulating tubule to reduce reabsorption of water

A. Assertion-true, reason-false B. Assertion-false, reason true
C. Both are true D. Both are false

449. A 30 -years old patient presented with episodic HT and headache, with a thyroid nodule. The investigation of choice is :

A. Urinary 5 - HIAA
B. Urinary catecholamines + aspiration of nodule
C. Thyroid hormone estimation
D. Thyroid Scan

450. Glycosolated hemoglobin percentage which indicates good control of diabetes :

A. 8% B. 10%
C. 15% D. 20%

451. In primary hyperaldosteronism following are true, except :

A. Edema B. Muscular weakness
C. HT D. Polyuria

452. Life long treatment is necessary in :

A. Myxoedema B. Addison's disease
C. Juvenile diabetes D. All of the above

453. The hormone responsible for the changes seen in phaeochromocytoma is :

A. Norepinephrine B. Thyroxine
C. Glucagon D. Serotonin
E. 5-hydroxytryptophan

454. A young diabetic has weight loss and hyperglycaemia but is not prone to ketoacidosis. He does not have pancreatic calculi. He is most likely to be a case of :

A. IDDM B. Diabetes with malnutrition
C. NIDDM D. Diabetes due to casava

455. Which of the following indicates secondary thyrotoxicosis :

A. Thyroid swelling B. Increased thyroglobulin
C. Increased TSH D. Increased T3

456. Thyroid crisis is common in :

A. Thyroid surgery
B. I131 administration
C. Administration of β-blockers
D. All of the above

Ans.	448.A	449.B	450.A	451.A	452.D	453.A
	454.C	455.C	456.A			

457. In hyperparathyrodism, which of the following is correct ?

A. Lower serum calcium
B. High serum calcium and low phosphorus
C. High serum calcium and high phosphorus
D. None of the above

458. 'Somogyi effect' is :

A. Ketosis induced insulin resistance
B. Hyperglycaemia and ketosis produced by counter-regulatory hormones
C. Paradoxical hypoglycaemia after glucose load
D. Inability to appreciate symptoms of hypoglycaemia

459. None metastatic endocrine manifeations are seen in :

A. Oat cell carcinoma
B. Hypernephroma
C. Wilm's tumour
D. Phaeochromocytoma

460. The features of inappropriate ADH secretion are except :

A. Hyponatraemia and hypochloraemia
B. Urinary sodium reflecting intake
C. Normal renal function
D. Normal adrenal function
E. None of the above

461. In patients with adrenal-cortical hyperplasia the treatment of choice is :

A. Total bilateral adrenalectomy
B. Unilateral partial adrenalectomy
C. Unilateral total adrenalectomy
D. Pituitary irradiation

462. The symptoms of endemic goitre include all, except :

A. Enlargement of thyroid gland
B. Dysphagia
C. Hoarseness
D. Heat intolerance
E. Cold intolerance

463. c-GMP is the second messenger for :

A. Insulin
B. Thyroxin
C. GH
D. FSH

464. The most common cause of hypothyroidism in the adult is :

A. Antithyroid chemicals
B. Parathyroid surgery
C. Radioactive iodine ingestion
D. Primary hypothyroidism

Ans. **457.B** **458.C** **459.A** **460.E** **461.A** **462.D** **463. A** **464. D**

465. Extragenital signs of gonadal-dysgenesis include all, except :
A. Aplasia of muscles B. Low set ears
C. Short stature D. Long spindly fingers

466. Most common cause of hypoparathyroidism is :
A. End organ resistance B. Surgical removal
C. Familial D. Idiopathic

467. Adrenal reserve is best tested by means of infusion with :
A. Glucocorticoids B. ACTH
C. Glucagon D. Metyrapone

468. Most probable diagnosis in a 42 year male with enlarged aeral parts, coarsening of facial features, and arthrlgias is :
A. Hypercorticism B. Acromegaly
C. Hypothyrodism D. Hypoparathyrodism

469. One of the following does not cause worsening of diabetes mellitus :
A. High carbohydrate meal
B. Infection
C. Acute anxiety
D. Hypoadrenalism
E. Increased production of human GH

470. Growth hormone causes following except :
A. Glycogen deposition B. Neoglucogenesis
C. Prevents protein catabolism D. Ketogenes

471. Following are features of diabetes insipidus, except :
A. Polyuria & Polydipsia
B. Specific gravity of urine is about 1002-1004
C. It contains sugar
D. Urine is clear
E. It does not contain protein

472. Prediabetic state can be diagnosed with certainly in :
A. Nondiabetic identical twin of diabetic mother
B. Offspring of diabetic parents
C. Obese relative of a diabetic
D. Brother of a diabetic male

473. Galactorrhea may be associated with the use of the following drugs except ;
A. Methyldopa B. Tricyclic antidepressants
C. Pyridoxine D. Phenothiazine

474. Sheehan's syndrome occurs after :
A. Head injury B. Hypothalmic trauma
C. Craniopharyngioma D. Suprasellar aneurysm
E. Postpartum haemorrhage

Ans.	465.D	466.B	467.B	468.B	469.D	470.A
	471.C	472.A	473. C	474. E		

475. Adrenalicalcification is a feature of all except :

A. Cushing's syndrome
B. Wollman's syndrome
C. Addison's syndrome
D. Neuroblastoma

476. Which of the following is wrong :

	Calcium	PO4	Alkaline Phosphatase
A. Hyper parathyrodism	↑	↓	↑
B. Rickets of Osteomalacia	↓	↑	↓
C. Paget's disease of bone	normal	normal	↑
D. Osteoporosis	normal	normal	↑

477. Hypertension is invariably associated with :

A. Acromegaly
B. Nelson's syndrome
C. Conn's syndrome
D. Klinefelter's syndrome

478. In Addison's disease :

A. There is always low serum sodium
B. Detected by pigmentation
C. Pallor always seen
D. Autoimmunity is the commonest cause

479. Best treatment of diabetic ketoacidosis is :

A. 3 hourly soluble insulin
B. 6 hourly soluble insulin
C. Large bolus subcutaneously
D. Slow infusion of soluble insulin

480. Enzyme deficient in diabetes mellitus is :

A. Glucokinase
B. Hexokinase
C. Phosphorylase
D. Pyrophosphate dehydrogenase

481. Which is not a feature of hypothyroidism :

A. Myxedemia
B. Carpal tunnel syndrome
C. Menorrhagia
D. Increased appetite

482. SIADH is seen in all except :

A. Oat cell carcinoma
B. Acute intermittent prophyria
C. Vincristine therapy
D. Primary pulmonary emphysema

Ans.	475.A	476.D	477.A	478.A	479.D	480.A
	481.D	482.D				

483. The characteristic and common neurological presentation of diabetes mellitus is :

A. Mononeuropathy
B. Symmetrical sensory polyneuropathy
C. Autonomic neuropathy
D. Cranial nerve palsies

484. Long acting thyroid stimulant is :

A. IgM B. IgG
C. IgD D. IgA

485. True about thyrotoxicosis is :

A. May come in remissions
B. Eye changes are always present
C. Cardiac changes are always present
D. Iodine deficiency is the commonest cause

486. Long administration of ACTH produces :

A. Osteoporosis B. Osteochondritis
C. Calcification of cartilage D. Osteopetrosis

487. A patient with asthenia ↓ BP, buccal pigmentation, ↑ Serum calcium has :

A. Hyperthyroidism B. Addison's disease
C. Cushing's syndrome D. Niacin deficiency

488. Definite diagnosis of diabites mellitus is :

A. Glycosuria
B. Glycosuria +Ketosis
C. Ketosis
D. Post prandial sugar > 180 mg%

489. Thyrotoxicosis can be best differentiated from anxiety neurosis clinically by :

A. Tachycardia B. Sleeping pulse rate
C. Moist hands D. Ankle jerk

490. Gigantism and acromegaly is because of :

A. ↑ TSH B. ↑ ACTH
C. ↑ Somatotrophin D. ↓ GH

491. Decrease in ADH secretion is caused by :

A. Thiazides B. Caffeine
C. Alcohol D. Vitamin C

492. hyperosmolar non-ketotic coma can be precipitated in a diabetic patient by :

A. Propranolol B. Phenytoin
C. Phenformin D. Metformin

Ans.	483.A	484.B	485.A	486.A	487.B	488.B
	489.B	490.C	491.C	492.C		

493. Virilisation of females is present in all of the following except :

A. 21 β-hydroxylase deficiency
B. 11 β-hydroxylase deficiency
C. 12 β-hydroxylase deficiency
D. 17 α-hydroxylase deficiency

494. Which of the following decreases insulin secretion ?

A. Growth Hormone
B. Glucocorticoids
C. Epinephrine
D. Glucose

495. Hypothermia can be seen in :

A. Hyperthyroidism
B. Myxoedema
C. Hyperparathyroidism
D. Goitre with Euthyroid status

496. Myxoedema coma is treated with :

A. Hydrocortisone
B. IV fluids
C. T3 injections
D. All of the above

497. Unpleasant flushingof face (Disulfiram-like) occurs with alcohol if taken along with :

A. Tolbutamide
B. Glibenclamide
C. Chlorpropamide
D. Metoformin

498. Consider the following statements regarding human insulin :

1. It is obtained from human pancreas
2. It differs from bovine insulin by three amino acids
3. It is more likely to cause lipo-atrophy
4. It is much less antigenic than bovine insulin

Of these statements

A. 1 and 3 are correct
B. 2 and 3 are correct
C. 1,2 and 4 are correct
D. 2 and 4 are correct

499. Insulin should not be given in :

A. Juvenile diabetes mellitus
B. Diabetes mellitus with infection
C. Sulfonylurea failure
D. Renal glycosuria

500. Raised thyroxine in pregnancy is because of :

A. ↑ Binding proteins
B. ↑ Synthesis
C. ↑ Release
D. Goitrogens

501. A young female with serum calcium lavel 11.5 gm%, Phosphate - 2.5 gm%, Alkaline PO4- 30 IU/L, Bony pains and muscular weakness, Correct diagnosis is :

A. Primary hyperparathyrodism
B. Secondary hyperparathyroidism

Ans.	493.D	494.C	495.B	496.D	497.C	498.C
	499.D	500.A	501.A			

C. Osteomalacia
D. Rickets

502. Biochemical abnormalities in the primary aldosteronism :
A. Potassium less than 3.5 mEq/L
B. Chlorides less than 95 mEq/L
C. HCO3 more than 30 mEq/L
D. All of the above

503. Abdominal complications of diabetes mellitus include each of the following except :
A. Appendicits
B. Ulcer perforation
C. Peritonitis
D. Henoch-Schonlein purpura

504. In a women between 15-35 years, the Cushing's syndrome shows following features, except :
A. Moon shaped plethoric face
B. Fuffalo type obesity
C. Hypotension
D. Amenorrhoea

505. Spot the "forbidden food" in management of diabetes mellitus :
A. Meat
B. Rice
C. Tea/Coffee
D. Spinach

506. Sexual complications of diabetes mellitus include each of the following except :
A. Precocious puberty
B. Reduction of fertility
C. Early menopause
D. None of the above

507. ACTH-dependent causes of Cushing's syndrome include each of the following except :
A. Iatrogenic
B. Adenomas or carcinomas of adrenal cortex
C. Pituitary-dependent bilateral adrenocortical hyperplasia, conventionally called Cushing's disease
D. Ectopic ACTH syndrome i.e secretion of ACTH by malignant or benign tumours of non-endocrine origin

508. Features of idiopathic hypoparathyroidism include each of the following except :
A. Tetany
B. Psychosis
C. Cataracts
D. Papilledema
E. Hepatosplenomegaly

509. Von Recklinghausen's disease results due to all of the following except :
A. Adenoma of parathyroid
B. Carcinoma of parathyroid
C. Hyperplasia of parathyroid
D. Surgical removal of parathyroid

Ans.	502.D	503.D	504.C	505.B	506.A	507.B
	508.E	509.D				

W510. **Low serum phosphate level (below 3 mg%) are seen in all of the following except :**

A. Fanconi's syndrome B. Hyperparathyroidism
C. Osteomalacia D. Rickets

511. **The specific lesion of diabetic retinopathy is :**

A. Hard exudate B. Microaneurysm
C. Retinal Haemorrhage D. Preretinal Haemorrhage

512. **Relative risk of developing I.D.D.M. is highest with HLA :**

A. DW4DR4 B. DW3DR3
C. DW3DR4 D. DW2DR2

513. **Hyperglycemia occurs when about what % of β cell mass is destroyed :**

A. 40% B. 60%
C. 80% D. 90%

514. **Consider the following conditions :**

1. Diabetic ketoacisosis 2. Prolonged fasting
3. Alcohol inotoxication 4. Hyperosmolar coma

Ketonuria is a feature of

A. 2 and 3 B. 1 and 2
C. 1,3 and 4 D. 1,2 and 3

515. **Kimmelstiel-Wilson bodies are characteristic of :**

A. Amyloidosis
B. Diabetic Nephropathy
C. Systemic lupus Erythematosus
D. Malignant Hypertension

516. **The earliest lesion of diabetic retinopathy is :**

A. Microaneurysm
B. Capillary dilatation and closure
C. Hard exudate
D. Haemorrhage

517. **Plasma T3 is increased in :**

A. Thyrotoxicosis B. Myxoedema
C. Addison's disease D. Hypopituitarism

518. **Simmond's disease manifests as following except :**

A. Acute onset of adult B. Asthenia
C. Accelerated metabolic rate D. Loss of sexual functions

519. **The causes of gangrene in diabetes include, all except :**

A. Infection B. Vasospasm
C. Perpheral neuritis D. Elevated blood sugar levels

Ans.	510.NONE	511.A	512.C	513.D	514.D	515.B
	516.A	517.A	518. C	519. B		

520. "Hour-glass" vertebrae and "triradiate pelvis" are seen radiologically in :

A. Thyrotoxicosis
B. Myxoedema
C. Cretinism
D. Hyperparathyroidism

521. Wasting of muscles in severe diabetes is due to :

A. Gluconeogenesis from proteins of tissues
B. Polyuria
C. Loss of vitamins
D. All of the above

522. A 55 year old female with generalized hyper-pigmentation and BP-80/60 mm Hg has :

A. Thyrotoxicosis
B. Myxoedma
C. Alkaptonuria
D. Addison's disease

523. Porphobilinogen is found in urine of patients with :

A. Hepatic cutanea tarda
B. Cutanea tarda
C. Erythropoitic porphyria
D. Intermittent acute porphyria

524. Diabetes mellitus occurs in all, except :

A. Amyloidosis
B. Large pancreatic cyst
C. Haemochromatosis
D. Cancer of pancreas

525. Recognised features of hyperparathyroidism include except :

A. Normal alkaline phosphatase
B. Reduction in hypercalcaemia after hydrocortisone
C. Hyperphospaturia
D. Increased blood urea
E. Increased urinary hydroxyproline

526. A 35-year old male with a history of renal calculi is seen because of polyuria and polydipsia. Urine examination reveals sp. gr. of 1008 and calcium oxalate crystals on microscopic examination. X-ray of KUB region reveals nephrocalcinosis. The most likely diagnosis is :

A. Polycystic renal disease
B. Hypoparathyroidism
C. Hyperparathyroidism
D. Diabetes insipidus

527. Adrenal steroid therapy may be useful in all of the following diseases, except :

A. Chronic sarcoidosis
B. Hamman-Rich syndrome
C. Pulmonary alveolar proteinosis
D. Goodpasture's syndrome

Ans.	520. D	521. A	522. D	523. D	524. A	525. B
	526. C	527. C				

528. **Central Diabetes Insipidus is characterised by :**
A. Low plasma and low urine osmilaity
B. High plasma and high urine osmilality
C. Low plasma and high urine osmilality
D. Low urine and high plasma osmilality

529. **To monitor therapy response in hypothyroidism, best is :**
A. T3
B. T4
C. TSH
D. r T3

530. **Which one of the following statements regarding non-insulin dependent diabetes mellitus (NIDDM) is not correct?**
A. Hyperinsulinaemia is frequent
B. Insulin resistance is common
C. Hypoinsulinaemia is always present
D. Hypoinsulinaemia may be seen only in late stages

531. **NIDDM is characterized by following except :**
A. Obesity
B. Ketoacidosis
C. Age of onset above 40
D. Insulin normal or high

532. **Recognised features of Hashimoto's disease include :**
A. High titre of thyroid autoantibodies
B. Exophthalmos
C. Hypothyroidism
D. Presence of parietal cell antibodies
E. Enlargement of the goitre when 1-thyroxine is given

533. **Investigation of a case of hypothyroidism due to primary involvement of the thyroid gland may show :**
A. No rise to TSH in response to intravenous TRH
B. An abnormally low ESR
C. Reduced thyroid binding globulin
D. Increased creatinine phosphokinase
E. Delta waves on EEG

534. **All are features of hypoglycemia, except :**
A. Brisk reflexes
B. Extensor plantar response
C. Bounding pulse
D. Low plasma bicarbonate
E. Normal or raised blood pressure

535. **Adenomas in Parathyroid are most often located in :**
A. Superior parathyroid
B. Inferior parathyroid
C. Thymus
D. Thyroid

Ans.	528. A	528. C	530. C	531. B	532. E	533. D
	534. D	535. B				

536. $K^+$is 1.6 meq/L. Diagnosis is :

A. Cushing's syndrome B. Conn's syndrome
C. Phaeochromocytoma D. ARF

537. The residual form of pheochromocytoma is treated by :

A. Strontium B. Phosphorus
C. I^{131} D. MIBG

538. Glucocorticoids are contraindicated in the following except :

A. Organ transplant B. Peptic ulcer
C. Hypertension D. Diabetes mellitus

539. In a 60-year old female with polydypsia, water deprivation test was performed and the values obtained are as follows :

Baseline	After vasopressin
Na-139 meq/L	Na—142 meq/L
K—3.6 meq/L	K—3.9 meq/L
Osm. Plasma—274 mosm/L	Plasma osm.—271 mosm/L
Osm. urine—150	Urine osm. —489 mosm/L

These findings suggest a diagnosis of :

A. Cranial DI B. Psychogenic polydypsia
C. Nephrogenic DI D. SIADH

540. A 60-year old female with history of depres-sion underwent radical mastectomy for Ca breast presented 6 weeks later with polyuria and polydypsia. Serum electrolytes —Na 139 meq/L, Ca-9.5 mg%, Most likely diagnosis is :

A. Hypercalciuria B. Diabetes insipidus
C. Psychogenic polydypsia D. Diabetes mellitus

541. Which of the following is not an indication for operation in nodular non toxic goitre ?

A. Oesophageal or Tracheal obstruction
B. Development of toxic goitre
C. Danger of development of thyroiditis
D. Danger of carcinomatous degeneration

542. Which one of the following statements about non- insulin dependent diabetes mellitus (NIDDM) is not true ?

A. Circulating islet cell antibodies are usually found
B. There is no HLA association
C. Ketosis is rare
D. Relative resistance to insulin is present

Ans. 536. B 537. D 538. C 539. C 540. C 541. C 542. A

543. **In progressive hypopituitarism of the following the first to stop being secreted is :**

A. T.S.H.	B. A.C.T.H
C. A.D.H	D. F.S.H. and L.H.
E. S.T.H.

544. **Features of Pickwickian syndrome may include :**

A. Obesity	B. Somnolence
C. Polycythaemia	D. Hypercapnia
E. All of the above

545. **Chronic Hashimoto's thyroiditis presents as :**

A. Hyperthyroidism	B. Hypothyroidism
C. Tracheal obstruction	D. Mass in the neck
E. Carcinoma of the neck

546. **Common symptoms (affecting 25% or more of patients) of phaeochromocytoma include following except :**

A. Headache	B. Palpitations
C. Sweating	D. Fear
E. Severe weight loss

547. **Loss of weight is a characteristic feature of :**

A. Hypothalamic lesions	B. Cushing's syndrome
C. Thyrotoxicosis	D. Myxoedema

548. **Adrenogenital syndrome is characterized by in- creased excretion of ——— in urine :**

A. 17 ketosteroids	B. 17-oxysteroids
C. Epiandrotestosterone	D. VMA

549. **Most specific and reliable test for Addison's disease is :**

A. 8 hour I.V. Cortisol test	B. Urinary VMA
C. Urinary 17 ketosteroids	D. Blood ACTH level

550. **Which of the following antidiabetic drugs are particularly to be avoided in elderly diabetic patients ?**

1. Glibenclamide	2. Gliclazide
3. Chlorpropamide	4. Glipizide

Select the correct answer using the codes given below :

Codes :

A. 1 and 2	B. 1 and 3
C. 2 and 4	D. 1,3 and 4

551. **Immunosupressed diabetics in ketoacidosis appear to be particularly susceptible to which of the following mycosis :**

A. Blastomycosis	B. Zygomycosis
C. Sporotrichosis	D. Rhinosporodiosis

Ans.	543. E	544. E	545. B	546. E	547. C	548. A
	549. A	550. B	551. B			

552. A high plasma calcitonin level causes :
A. Bone demineralization
B. Increased formation of 25 dihydroxy cholecalciferol
C. Decreased blood coagulability
D. Increased formation of 24-25 dihydroxy cholecalciferol

553. The following is true of untreated panhypopitiuitarism :
A. Pigmentation of skin
B. Mineralocorticoid deficiency
C. Glucocosticoid deficiency
D. Gonadal atrophy

554. Which of the following symptom excludes hyperaldo-steronism
A. Hypokalemia B. Hypernatremia
C. Albuminuria D. Malignant HT

555. Congenital malformation of fetus in diabetic mother is diagnosed by :
A. Serum AFP B. Amniotic fluid AFP
C. Fructosamine serum level D. HbA1AC

556. In ectopic ACTH due to small Ca lung, seen in :
A. Hyperpigmentation is unusual
B. Typical cushingoid habitus seen
C. Dexamethasone 8 mg orally suppresses cortisol
D. Hypokalemic alkalosis

557. Diagnostic criteria for impaired thyroglobulin syntheisis include all, except :
A. Presence of colloid spaces B. Low radioiodine uptake
C. Hypothyroid D. Goiter

558. Failure of renal tubules to respond to exogenous parathonone is seen in :
A. Post radiation hypoparathyroidism
B. Post surgical hypoparathyroidism
C. Pseudohypoparathyroidism
D. Pseudopseudohypoparathyrodism

559. Paradoxical GH increases with administration of TSH in following except :
A. Acromegaly B. Prolactinemia
C. Malnutrition D. Anorexia nervosa

560. Hypertriglyceridemia is commonly seen in :
A. Nephrotic syndrome B. Abetalipoproteinemia
C. LDL receptor defect D. Dysbetalipoproleinemia

Ans.	552. D	553. C	554. C	555. D	556. D	557. B
	558. C	559. B	560. A			

561. **Obstructive Azoospermia is present in :**
A. William's Campbell syndrome
B. Mounier Khan syndrome
C. Young's syndrome
D. Yellow nail syndrome

562. **Diagnosis of adrenal insufficiency in the absence of crisis depends upon :**
A. Reduction in a plasma 17-hydroxy corticoids and its failure to rise after corticotrophin
B. Lack of increase in urinary excretion of 17-keto and 11-hydroxysteroids after corticotrophin
C. Lack of adequate increase in urine volume after water load test
D. Increase in Na/K ratio above 2.0 in saliva
E. Any of the above

563. **Methimazole interfers with thyroid function mainly by :**
A. Inhibition of thyroidal organic binding and coupling reactions
B. Destruction of thyroid cells
C. Immunological means
D. Inhibition of iodine uptake

564. **Minimum amount of carbohydrate required to prevent ketonuria in a case of diabetes is about :**
A. 50 gm/daily
B. 25 gm/daily
C. 100 gm/daily
D. 150 gm/daily
E. 200 gm/daily

565. **Following are features of myxoedema, except :**
A. Marked slowing of the recovery phase of ankle jerk
B. Speech is slow, monotonous and croaking in character
C. Thin lips, small tongue with puffy eyelids
D. Sparse, short and lustureless hairs
E. Pulse in slow

566. **In patients with myxoedema the administration of thyroxine is followed by :**
A. A diuresis and an initial rapid and marked fall in weight
B. An increase in the weight
C. Oliguria
D. B+C

567. **In a case of adrenal insufficiency, a sudden exacerebation may be precipitated by :**
A. A mild infection
B. Chilling
C. Fasting
D. Diarrhoea
E. All of the above

Ans. **561. C** **562. E** **563. A** **564. C** **565. C** **566. A** **567. E**

568. Which of the following is frequently an early complaint, giving warning of an impending crisis in a case of adrenal insufficiency :

A. Epigastric pain
B. Severe vomiting
C. Hypotension
D. Pyrexia
E. Weakness and tiredness

569. The serum PBI concentration is affected by all, except :

A. A myelogram five years previously
B. Administration of oestrogen containing contraceptive pills
C. Di-iodohyroxyquinolines
D. Administration of spironolactone

570. Most useful test in diabetes mellitus is :

A. Urine sugar
B. Glycosylated Haemoglobin
C. Glucose tolerance test
D. Post prandial blood sugar

571. In myxoedema the patient complains of :

A. Palpitations
B. Tremors
C. Weight loss
D. Eructation
E. Intolerance of cold

572. Acromegaly occurs most frequently in :

A. Childhood
B. Adolescents
C. Adults
D. Middle-aged
E. Elderly

573. Insulin resistance is said to be existing when the daily dose of insulin increases :

A. > 100 IU
B. > 150 IU
C. > 200 IU
D. > 300 IU
E. > 500 IU

574. Which of the following may be related to hypothyroidism?

A. Congenital deafness
B. 'J' Waves on the ECG
C. Low serum B12
D. All of the above
E. None of the above

575. True about azotemic psuedo diabetes is :

A. Decreased sensitivity of peripheral tissues to insulin
B. Normal serum glucose & increased urinary glucose
C. Decreased insulin levels
D. Renal glycosuria

576. Feature of thyroid eye disease includes all, except :

A. Conjunctival irritation
B. Corneal oedema
C. Extraocular muscles infiltered with lymphocytes
D. Herniation of orbital fat into the eyelids

Ans. 568. A 569. D 570. C 571. E 572. D 573. A 574. D 575. A 576. B

577. **Which of the following is not an antithyroid drug ?**
A. Propranolol
B. Propyl thiouracil
C. Potassium perchlorate
D. Carbimazole

578. **'Pointed' facies may be seen in :**
A. Hypothyroidism
B. G H deficiency
C. Bone-cartilage dysplasia
D. Russell-silver dwarfism

579. **In primary haemochromatosis, all are seen except :**
A. Chorea
B. Diabetes mellitus
C. Cirrhosis of liver
D. Arthritis

580. **Tetany is caused by all except :**
A. Thyroid surgery
B. Hyperventilation
C. Verapamil
D. Malabsorption

581. **Phosphate diabetes - mode of inheritance :**
A. Autosomal recessive
B. Autosomal dominant
C. X-linked recessive
D. X-linked dominant

582. **Estimation of glycosylate hemoglobin gives an assessment of the blood glucose level in the previous ——— weeks :**
A. 1
B. 2
C. 8
D. 12

583. **Which of the following is false about diabetic keto acidosis :**
A. Low dose insulin therapy is given
B. Leucocytosis suggests infection
C. Pyrexia is unusual even if there is infection
D. Dehydration out of proportion to severity of vomiting

584. **Heel pad thickness is useful in :**
A. Hypothyroidism
B. Acromegaly
C. PEM
D. Hypogonadism

585. **HLA linkage is seen in :**
A. IDDM
B. NIDDM
C. Secondary diabetes due to pancreatic disease
D. Diabetes due to insulin antagonist

586. **The laboratory test of choice in myxoedema coma is :**
A. Thyroid stimulating hormone (TSH)
B. Thyrotropin releasing hormone (TRH)
C. Tri-idiothyronine (T3)
D. Tetra-iodothyronine (T4)

587. **Which one of the following is not associated with cataract ?**
A. Galactosaemia
B. Prolonged coticosteroid therapy
C. Hypoparathyroidism
D. Magnesium excretion

Ans.						
	577. A	**578. D**	**579. A**	**580. C**	**581. D**	**582. D**
	583. A	**584. B**	**585. A**	**586. D**	**587. D**	

588. Activation of the renin stimulates :
A. Water excretion
B. Potassium retention
C. Sodium retention
D. Magnesium excretion

589. Glucagon stimulates all of the following except :
A. Glycogenolysis
B. Bile secretion
C. Hydrochloric acid secretion
D. Intestinal secretion

590. Which of the following pituitary tumour produces enamel :
A. Meningioma
B. Chordoma
C. Teratoma
D. Craniopharyngioma

591. The commonest complication of diabetes mellitus is :
A. KW syndrome
B. Necrotizing papillitis
C. UTI
D. Kidney failure

592. ↓ TBG (Thyroid bound globulin) is seen in :
A. Nephrotic syndrome
B. Pregnancy
C. Billiary cirrhosis
D. Oral contraceptive
E. Acute intermittent porphyria

593. Hypoaldosteronism with low urine Na+ is seen in all except :
A. Severe gastroenteritis
B. Severe CCF
C. SIA diabetes mellitus
D. Duodenal fistula
E. Chronic diarrhoea

594. Hyperplasia of parathyroid glands is seen in follwing except :
A. Malabsorption syndrome
B. Chronic renal failure
C. Vitamin D deficiency
D. Sarcoidosis

595. In myxedema, which is not correct :
A. Slow pulse
B. Hypertension
C. Hypotension
D. Dry skin

596. Hypoglycemia in full term infant is defined when blood sugar is less than :
A. 70 mg%
B. 60 mg%
C. 30 mg%
D. 20 mg%

597. Berry's sign is present in :
A. Retrosternal goitre
B. Carcinoma thyroid
C. Grave's disease
D. Ca head of Pancreas

598. Hypoglycaemia is not seen in :
A. Sarcoma
B. Hepatoma
C. Small cell Ca
D. Mesothelioma

Ans.	588. C	589. C	590. D	591. C	592. A	593. B
	594. D	595. C	596. C	597. B	598. C	

599. Gynaecomastia can be caused by the intake of all of the following drugs, except :

A. Ethionamide B. Isoniazid
C. Methyl Dopa D. Streptomycin

600. Galactorrhoea can occur in all of the following except :

A. Prolactinomas
B. Ectopic productin of HPL lactogen and prolactin
C. Hyperthyroidism
D. Reserpine therapy

601. Which bone condition is associated with endocrine disturbance :

A. Chondroma B. Osteoma
C. Fibrous dysplasia D. Osteochondromas

602. Grave's disease may be associated with all except :

A. Addison's disease B. Hoshimoto's disease
C. Vitiligo D. Polymyositis

603. Oral hypoglycemics are useful in diabetes mellitus of :

A. Mild stable maturity onset type
B. Juvenile type
C. Diabetes who is obese
D. Diabetic ketoacidosis type

604. G subunit deficiency is seen in Pseudohypo-parathyroidism type :

A. Ia B. Ib
C. II D. All of the above

605. In Addison's disease, untrue is :

A. Always low sodium levels
B. Detected by pigmentation of skin
C. Hypertension
D. Autoimmune phenomenon is the commonest cause

606. Which hormone deficiency in hypopituitarism is not treated in adults :

A. ACTH B. Thyroxine
C. GH D. Gonadotrophins

607. 1 Unit of insulin neutalizes :

A. 1.0 gm of glucose B. 2.5 gm of glucose
C. 4 gm of glucose D. 5 gm of glucose

608. True about secretions by adrenal is :

	Zona glomerulosa	Zona reticularis	Zona fasciculata
A.	Aldosterone	Androgen	Corticosteroid
B.	Corticosteroids	Androgen	Aldosterone
C.	Androgen	Aldosteron	Corticosteroids
D.	Aldosterone	Cortico-steroids	Androgen

Ans.	599. D	600. C	601. C	602. D	603. A	604. A
	605. C	606. C	607. B	608. A		

609. 24 hours excretion of cortisol is approximately :

A. 5 mg B. 10 mg
C. 20 mg D. 30 mg

610. Hypoglycemia is found in :

A. Insulin over dose B. Hypopituitarism
C. Adrenocortical tumour D. All of the above

611. Features of hyperthyroidism are :

A. Pericardial effusion B. Menorrhagia
C. Delayed ankle relaxation D. Heat intolerance

612. Which of the following is mainly mineralocorticoid :

A. Prednislone B. Dexamethasone
C. DOCA D. Hydrocortisone

613. Diabetic retinopathy is related to :

A. Duration of disease B. Severity of disease
C. Family history D. Control of diabetes

614. Which of the following is not a treatment of Grave's disease :

A. I^{131} B. Propranolol
C. Subtotal thyroidectomy D. Medium thyroidectomy

615. Beta endorphins are released from :

A. Thyroid
B. Posterior lobe of the pituitary
C. Anterior and intermediate lobe of pituitary
D. Adrenal cotex

616. A metabolite of androgenic hormone is :

A. 17-OH steroid B. 17 ketosteroid
C. 17 ketogenic steroid D. Pragantriol

617. Thyroid storm is due to excessive secretion of :

A. TSH B. Thyroxine
C. Catechloaemines D. Steroids

618. In diabetic ketoacidosis, correct is :

A. Low serum potassium B. Increased ion gap
C. Metabolic alkalosis D. Respiratory acidosis

619. Fungal lung infection commonly seen in diabetics is :

A. Actinomycosis B. Mucormycosis
C. Aspergillosis D. Coccidiodomycosis

Match the following :

A. Outward appearance of acromegaly but has clubbing, periosteal thickening
B. Sexual infantilism, adiposity
C. Adiposity, polydactyly, genital atrophy, mental retardation
D. Persistent postpartum lactation and amenorrhea

Ans.	609. C	610. D	611. D	612. C	613. A	614. D
	615. C	616. D	617. B	618. B	619. B	

620. **Chiari-Frommel syndrome :**

621. **Idiopathic hypertrophic osteoarthropathy :**

622. **Laurence - Moon - Biedl - syndrome :**

623. **Frohlich's syndrome :**

624. **Which of the following if present would rule out Hyperaldosteronism :**
A. Elevated serum sodium level
B. Periodic paralysis
C. Albuminuria
D. Malignant hypertension

625. **The peak blood sugar level following a standard oral GTT occurs normally at :**
A. 30 minutes
B. 60 minutes
C. 90 minutes
D. 120 minutes

626. **A primary hypothyroid patient presents in summer month with features of neurological obturation and behaviour abnormality. The most appropriate investigation would be :**
A. Thyroxine
B. Glucose
C. Creatinine
D. Sodium

627. **Which one of the followng statements about diabetes is not correct?**
A. Insulin may be given subcutaneously in patients of diabetic ketoacidosis
B. Insulin antibodies are a hallmark for diagnosis of insulin resistance
C. During hypoglycaemic episodes patient may complain of difficulty in vision
D. Urine may show positive test for ketone bodies for some time even after patients of diabetic ketosis are otherwise well controlled

628. **Acanthosis Nigricans is seen in :**
A. Addisons disease
B. Insulin resitance
C. Sarcoidosis
D. Amyloidosis

629. **All are true about glucose intolerance except :**
A. Estimation of FBS is essential for diagnosis
B. Diagnosis is usually done using FBS/PPBS
C. They cause macrovascular damage
D. None of the above

630. **A patient has hyperphosphatemia with short metacarpals and associated cataract.The diagnosis is :**
A. Pseudohypoparathyroidism
B. Hypophosphatesia
C. Hyperparathyroidism
D. Osteomalacia

Ans.	620. D	621. A	622. C	623. B	624. D	625. B
	626. D	627. A	628. B	629. D	630. A	

631. Fasting blood sugar level for diagnosis of diabetes mellitus is :

A. 114 mg/dl B. 120 mg/dl
C. 132 mg/dl D. 126 mg/dl

632. Calcitonin causes hypocalcemia by :

A. ↑ excretion by kidney B. ↓ bone resorption
C. ↓ absorbtion from gut D. PTH activity

633. Hyperphosphatemia, and hypocalcemia are seen in following except :

A. Hypoparathyroidism
B. CRF
C. Pseudo hypoparathyroidism
D. Malabsorbtion

634. Hyper calcemia is seen in the following except :

A. Vitamin D in toxication
B. Leukemia
C. Hyperproteinemia
D. Pseudohypoparathyroidism

635. An obese person presenting with fatigue had a blood glucose of 180mg%.The next step is:

A. Glycosylated Hb B. GIT
C. Fasting urine sugar D. None of the above

636. A patient with IDDM since 15 years. Most reliable early indicator of diabetic glomerulopathy is :

A. 0.12 gm - 0.15 gm albumin/day in 3 consecutive samples
B. 0.52 gm-0.64 gm of total proteins/day
C. Development of diabetic retinopathy
D. Development of diabetic neuropathy

637. A patient with vomiting presents with confusion. O/E Na 120 meq/LK-4.5 meq/L, oedema not seen, disease is :

A. Toxoplasmosis with SIADH
B. Liver cirrhosis
C. Severe dehydration
D. Viral encephalitis

638. A chronic alcoholic admitted with acute pancreatitis developed sudden blindness in the right eye after 3 days. The cause could be:

A. Alcohol withdrawal
B. Retinal vein thrombosis
C. Purtschener's retinopathy
D. Vitreous haemorrahage

Ans.	631. D	632. B	633. D	634. C	635. B	636. A
	637. A	638. C				

639. **68 year chandu is a diabetic and presented with black, foul smelling discharge from the nose. Examination revealed blackish discoloration of the inferior turbinate. The diagnosis is:**
A. Mucormycosis
B. Nasopharyngeal angiofibroma
C. Antrochoanal polyp
D. Foreign body

w640. **A 35 year old asymptomatic male was investigated and found to have hypercalcemia.He could be having:**
A. Primary hyperparathyroidism
B. Familial hypercalcuric hypercalcemia
C. Occult malignancy
D. Williams syndrome

641. **A 45 year old male presented with crectile impotence.Investigation showed a lowered testosterone level and a raised prolactin level.He has got:**
A. Cushing's syndrome B. Pituitary adenoma
C. Testicular failure D. Bromocriptine intake

642. **Following are the findings in hyperthyroidism except :**
A. Scratchy murmur at left heart border
B. Early diastolic murmur
C. Irreularly irregular pulse
D. Non ejection systolic click

643. **Hypoglycemia unawareness in diabetes is due to :**
A. Necrobiosis lipiodica B. Autonomic neuropathy
C. Insulin resistence D. Pancreatitis

644. **Commonest cause of thyroiditis :**
A. Autoimmune B. Riedel's
C. Hashimoto's D. Infection

645. **Hypoglycaemia is a common feature of all the following except :**
A. Sheehan's syndrome B. Insulinoma
C. Somatostatinoma D. Addison's disease

646. **Hypocalcaemia is a feature of all the following except :**
A. Chronic renal failure
B. Hypoparathyroidism
C. Pseudo-pseudohypoparathyroidism
D. Pseudo-hypoparathyroidism

647. **Diarrhoea in type II Diabetes mellitus is due to:**
A. Decreased absorptive power B. Imparied absorptive power
C. Decreased bile salt synthesis D. Decreased digestive power

Ans.	639. A	640. A,B	641. B	642. B	643. B	644. A
	645. C	646. C	647. B			

648. Which of the following is seen in hypopituitarism :

A. Pallor
B. ↓ BMR
C. Reduced response to stres
D. Cachexia

649. Commonest manifestation of cryptococous infection in AIDS is :

A. Pneumonitis
B. Meningitis
C. Hepatitis
D. Ophthalmitis

650. Insulin dose in IDDM nephropathy :

A. Increases
B. Decreases
C. Same
D. Oral antidiabetics are added

651. 30 years of young female presented with weakness, prominent of eye with increased T3 & T4 level with enlargement of thyroid seen in all except :

A. Diffuse enlargement of goitre
B. Adenomatous goitre
C. Reiel's struma
D. Hashimoto's-thyroiditis

652. "Hypoglycemia unawareness" in diabetes mellitus is due to :

A. Switch over insulin to oral drugs
B. Diabetic neuropathy
C. Insulin resistance
D. Necrobiosis lipoidica

653. Weight loss is seen in :

A. Cushing syndrome
B. Pheochromocytoma
C. Insulin secreting tumour
D. Hypothyroidism

654. Which is not true regarding apathetic hyperthyroidism :

A. Seen in elderly
B. Radioiodine treatment of choice
C. Cardiovascular manifestations are common
D. Inherited as Autosomal recessive

655. The most common hormone other than gastrin, contained in the gastrin-secreting islet cell tumour is :

A. ACTH
B. Glucagon
C. Melanocyte stimulating hormone
D. Growth hormone releasing factor
E. Insulin

656. About Cushing syndrome, true is :

A. Low dose dexamethasone suppress cortisone secretion
B. Ca of adrenal is more common than adenoma
C. Pituitory adenoma size > 2cm (usually)
D. ↑ ACTH secretion is the commonest cause

Ans.	648. D	649. B	650. C	651. D	652. B	653. B
	654. B	655. A	656. D			

657. **The drug of choice for very high circulatory catecholamine in phaeochromocytoma is :**

A. Phenoxybenzamine B. Prazosin
C. Doxazocin D. Propranolol

658. **Long term complications of steroid therapy include all the following except :**

A. Growth retardation B. Cataract
C. Potbelly D. Stress fractures

659. **Recombinant human insulin is made by :**

A. CDNA from any eukaryote cell
B. CDNA of pancreatic cell
C. Genome of any eukaryote
D. Genome of pancreatic cell

660. **Secondary hyperparathyroidism due to vit D deficiency shows :**

A. Hypocalcemia B. Hypercalcemia
C. Hyper phosphatemia D. Hypo phosphatemia

661. **Lalloo, 50 years old, a chronic smoker, presents with history of hemoptysis. He was having trunkal obesity and hypertension. He had an elevated ACTH level which was not suppressible with high dose dexamethasone. What would be the most probable diagnosis :**

A. Bilateral adrenal hyperplasia
B. Adrenal adenoma
C. Pituitary tumour
D. Ectopic ACTH producing lung cancer

662. **Starvation and diabetes mellitus can lead on to ketoacidosis. Which of the following features is in favour of ketoacidosis due to diabetes mellitus :**

A. Increase in glucagon/insulin ratio increased cAMP and increased blood glucose
B. Decreased insulin, increased free fatty acids which is equivalent to blood glucose
C. Decreased insulin, increased free fatty acids which is not equivalent to blood glucose
D. Elevated insulin and free fatty acid, equivalent to blood glucose

663. **A patient has an accident with resultant transection of the pituitary. What will not occur :**

A. Diabetes mellitus B. Diabetes insipidus
C. Hyperprolactinemia D. Hypothyroidism

Ans.	657. A	658. C	659. B	660. D	661. D	662. A
	663. A					

664. Most useful investigation in diabetic mother to identify DM in first pregnancy :

A. Glycosylated Hb B. GTT
C. ACTH levels D. Fasting and PP sugar

665. An obese person with weight 90 kgm was found to have blood sugar 490 mg% Ketone bodies was 1(+). Treatment of choice is :

A. Metformin B. Glibenclamide
C. Chlorpropamide D. Insulin

666. A 30-year old male complains of loss of erection with low testosterone and high prolactin level in blood. What is the likely diagnosis :

A. Pituitary disease B. Testicular failure
C. Cranio pharyngioma D. Cushing's syndrome

667. In a patient with cold intolerance, TSH low, T4 & T3 low, what is your diagnosis :

A. Pituitary failure B. Thyroprivic failure
C. Hypothalamic failure D. None

668. Prolactin content is highest in :

A. Pregnancy B. Pituitary adenoma
C. Premethazine therapy D. Sheehan's syndrome

669. A diabetic patient comes with diabetic ketoacidosis HCO3- is 12, condition is :

A. Metabolic acidosis with high HCO3-
B. Metabolic acidosis with low HCO3-
C. Metabolic alkalosis with low HCO3-
D. Metabolic alkalosis with high HCO3

670. Which of the following drugs is given intranasally for neuronal DI in both adults and children :

A. Desmopressin B. Pitressin
C. Beclamethasone D. Lypressin

671. Which porphyria presents with neuropsychiatric presentation normal colored urine and no skin lesions :

A. Porphyria cutanea tarda
B. a/c intermittent porphyria
C. Hereditary copro porhyria
D. Chester

672. The best investigation which is sensitive and specific for diagnosing neuroendocrine tumors in the body is :

A. Spiral CT scan B. Endoscopic ultrasound
C. Radiolabelled isotope scan D. PET scan

Ans.	664. A	665. D	666. A	667. A	668. B	669. B
	670. A	671. B	672. C			

673. **The following are features of Bartter's syndrome, except :**
A. Hypokalemia
B. Hypertension
C. Alkalosis
D. Increased renin and aldosterone

674. **Glucagonama is characterised by which of the following skin disorders ?**
A. Necrotising migratory erythema
B. Erythema chronium migrans
C. Erythema gyraturn repens
D. Acrodermatitis enteropathica

675. **The Benzoic acid derivative which stimulates insulin secretion during meats used in Rx of diabetes mellitus :**
A. Acarbose
B. Rosiglitazone
C. Repaglinide
D. Glimpride

676. **A patient with hyperparathyroidism with pheochromocytoma develops a thyroid swelling. This is most likely due to which of the following :**
A. Follicular adenoma
B. Papillary carcinoma
C. Medullary carcinoma
D. Follicular carcinoma

677. **True about Cushing's syndrome is :**
A. Adrenomedullary hypeplasia in associated with the MEN syndrome is a common cause
B. Bronchial carcinoid causes Cushings syndrome
C. It is diagnosed by hypokalemia in association with Increased adrenal secretion
D. It is often fatal due its coronary and Cerebrovascular accidents

678. **Tumor lysis syndrome does not lead to :**
A. Hypocalcemia
B. Hyperuricemia
C. Hypercalcemia
D. Hyperphosphatemia

679. **True about type II (NIDDM) diabetes mellitus :**
A. Increased level of insulin in serum
B. Ketoacidosis always present in untreated patients
C. B cells do not secrete insulin
D. Triglycerides level normal

680. **A 50 year old man presents with hemoptysis. ACTH level is increased and does not respond to dexamethasone suppression test. The most likely diagnosis is :**
A. Congenital adrenal hyperplasia
B. Ectopic ACTH production

Ans.	673. B	674. A	675. C	676. C	677. A	678. A
	679. A	680. B				

C. Cortical adrenal tumours
D. Miliary tuberculosis.

681. **A case of vitamin D resistant Rickets with calcium 9mg, phosphorus-2.4 mg and increased alkaline phosphatase. Most common cause is :**
A. Vitamin D dependant rickets
B. Renal tubular acidosis
C. Hypophasphatemic rickets
D. Hypoparathyroidism

682. **Glucose mediated release of insulin is mediated through :**
A. ATP dependent K channels
B. cAMP
C. Carrier modulation
D. Receptor phosphorylation

683. **All are true about de Quervain's thyroiditis except :**
A. Raised ESR
B. Subsides spontaneously
C. Autoimmune etiology
D. Pain and swelling of the thyroid occurs

684. **All the following statement about acute adrenal insufficiency are true except :**
A. Acute adrenal insufficiency is usually secondary to exogenous glucocorticoid administration
B. Hyperglycemia is usually present
C. Hyperkalemia may present as an acute cardiac problem.
D. Hypermatremia occurs as a result of renal tubule sodium reabsorption

685. **A 35 year old lady, Kamli, presenting with severe headache was found to have a thyroid nodule with ipssilateral enlarged cervical lymph nodes. She gave a history of her mother dying of thyroid cancer. Which of the following investigations should be done prior to surgery :**
A. Urinary metanephrine
B. Hydroxy indole acetic acid in urine
C. Urinary metanephrine and VMA
D. T3T4 and TSH

686. **In Pheochromocytoma all the following are seen except :**
A. Episodic hypertension
B. Orthostatic hypotension
C. Wheezing
D. Headache

687. **In Conn's syndrome, all the following are seen except :**
A. Hypokalemia
B. Hypermatremia
C. Hypertension
D. Edema

Ans. 681. C 682. A 683. C 684. B 685. C 686. C 687. D

688. **In which of the following conditions does hyperglycemia occur :**
A. Addison's disease B. Uremia
C. Acromegaly D. Fever

689. **TSH infusion test is used to detect :**
A. LH B. ACTH
C. GH reserve D. FSH

690. **Thyrotoxicosis with decreased radioactive iodine uptake is seen in :**
A. Grave's disease B. Toxic adenoma
C. De Quervain's thyroiditis D. Multinodular goitre

691. **Which of the following drug has best effect on lipid metabolism**
A. Propranolo B. Losartan
C. Prazosin D. Cholorothiazide

692. **Deficiency of growth hormone can be diagnosed by :**
A. Serum GH level B. Serum IGF-1 level
C. Insulin tolerance test D. GH response to clonidine

693. **A 25 year old young woman has recurrent episodes of headache and sweating. Her mother had renal calculi and died after having a neck mass. The physical examination reveals a thyroid nodule but not clinical sign of thyrotoxicosis. Before performing thyroid surgery, the surgeon should order :**
A. Measurement of thyroid hormones
B. Serial determinations of serum calcium, phosphorus, protein and alkaline phosphatase
C. 24-hours urine test for 5-hydroxyindoleacetic acid excretion
D. Serial 24 hours tests for catecholamines, metanephrines and vanillylmandelic acid excretion

694. **In DM type - II Insulin resistance develops due to :**
A. End organ target receptor insensitivity
B. DKA
C. HONK (Hyperosmolar nonketosis)
D. Genetic

695. **Consider the following statements :**
In nephrogenic diabetes insipidus the patient is likely to have :
1. High vasopressin level
2. Poor or no response to desmopressin
3. Low plasma osmolality
4. Elevated plasma glucose level

Which of these statements are correct :
A. 1, 2 and 3 B. 2, 3 and 4
C. 1 and 4 D. 1, 2 3 and 4

Ans.	688. C	689. B	690. C	691. C	692. C	693. D
	694. A	695. A				

696. Which one of the following features may not be seen in hypothyroidism :

A. Cold intolerance B. Deafness
C. Pericardial effusion D. Pretibial myxoedema

697. Consider the following statements :
In acromegaly the patient is likely to have

1. Impaired glucose tolerance
2. Galactorrhoea
3. Hypertension
4. Suppression of growth hormone with glucose

Which of these statements are correct :

A. 1,2 and 4 B. 2,3 and 4
C. 1, 3 and 4 D. 1, 2 and 3

698. Low serum sodium with normal serum osmolality is a feature of :

A. Primary polydipsia B. Diuretic use
C. Hyperlipidemia D. Hypoaldosteronism

699. A 30-year old male complains of infertility. He appears tall and has gynaecomastia. Genitalia appear normal except for bilateral small testes. His chromosomal pattern is likely to be :

A. 45 XO B. 47 XXY
C. 47 XYY D. 46 XY

700. All of the followng may occur in Noonan's syndrome except :

A. Hepertrophic cardiomyopathy
B. Cryptoorchidism
C. Infertility in females
D. Autosomal dominant transmission

701. A 45-year-old woman visited her physician with complaints of increased appetite and thirst with increased frequency of urination. She also had the symptoms of diminished or impalpable pulses in the feet, besides gangrene of the feet. Her laboratory findings on the oral glucose tolerance test are as follows:

Parameters	**Fasting**	**1 hour**	**2 hour**
Blood glucose (mg/dL)	155	270	205
Urine glucose	-ve	+++	++
Ketone bodies	-ve	-ve	-ve

Which of the following statements is not correct for the above mentioned case?

A. She was suffering from insulin dependent diabetes mellitus
B. She was suffering from non-insulin dependent diabetes mellitus
C. She was treated with oral hypoglycemic drugs only when diet control and exercise could not control the pathological situation
D. Knowledge of family history of diabetes mellitus is useful in predicting the nature of diabetes

Ans.	696. D	697. D	698. C	699. B	700. C	701. A

702. A 28 year old lady has put on weight (10 Kg over a period of 3 years), and has oligomenorrhoea followed by amenorrhoea for 8 months. The blood pressure is 160/100 mm of Hg. Which of the following is the most appropriate investigation?

A. Serum electrolytes
B. Plasma cortisol
C. Plasma testosterone and ultrasound evaluation of pelvis
D. T3, T4 and TSH

703. Estimation of the following hormones is useful while investigating a case of gynaecomastia except?

A. Testosterone
B. Prolactin
C. Estradiol
D. Luteinizing hormone

704. The occurence of hyperthyroidism following administration of supplemental iodine to subjects with endemic iodine deficiency goitre is known as?

A. Jod-Basedow effect
B. Wolff-Chaikoff effect
C. Thyrotoxicosis factitia
D. de Quervain's thyroiditis

705. The best marker to diagnose thyroid related disorders is?

A. T3
B. T4
C. TSH
D. Thyroglobulin

706. HBAic level in blood explains?

A. Acute rise of sugar
B. Long term status of blood sugar
C. Hepatorenal syndrome
D. Chronic pancreatitis

707. Which one of the following oral hypoglycemic agents is NOT an insulin secretogogue

A. Gliclazide
B. Glimiperide
C. Repaglinide
D. Rosiglitazone

708. A 50 year old male with type 2 diabetes mellitus is found to have 24 hr urinary albumium of 250 mg. Which of the following drugs may be used to retard progression of renal disease?

A. Hydrochlorothiazide
B. Enalapril
C. Amiloride
D. Aspirin

709. All of the following conditions are known to cause diabetes insipidus except :

A. Multiple sclerosis
B. Head injury
C. Histiocytosis
D. Viral encephalitis

710. The karyotype of a Patient with Androgen Insensitivity Syndrome is :

A. 4 xx
B. 46 xy.
C. 47 xxy
D. 45 x 0

Ans.	702. B	703. C	704. A	705. C	706. B	707. D
	708. B	709.A	710. B			

711. **Parcreatitis, pituitary tumor and phaeochromocytoma may be associated with :**
A. Medullary carcinoma of thyroid
B. Papillary carcinoma of thyroid
C. Anaplastic carcinoma of thyroid
D. Follicular carcinoma of thyroid

712. **Hypercalcemia associated with malignancy is most often mediated by :**
A. Parathyroid hormone (PTH)
B. Parathyroid hormone related protein (PTHrP).
C. Interleukin -6 (IL-6)
D. Calcitonin

713. **Which one of the following is true of adrenal suppression due to steroid therapy ?**
A. It is not associated with atrophy of the adrenal glands
B. It does not occur in patients receiving inhaling steroids
C. In should be expected in anyone receiving > 5 mg. Prednisolon daily
D. Following cessation, the stress response normalises after 8 weeks

714. **The classification proposed by the international Lymphoma Study Group for non-Hodgkin's lymphoma is known as :**
A. Kiel classification
B. REAL classification
C. WHO classification
D. Rappaport classification

715. **Commonest feature of hypoparathyroidism in children is :**
A. Catarac
B. Recurrent seizures
C. Cold extremities
D. Laryngospasm

716. **True about children with diabetes mellitus :**
A. Usually have an abrupt onset compared to adult onset
B. Should not be treated with oral hypoglycemic agents
C. Need not be concerned about developing renal eye complications at any time
D. Have marked variations in insulin response

717. **A newborn 7 days old with vomiting and dehydration. Clinical examination was normal except for hyperpigmentation of nipple. Serum electrolytes Na—120 meq/L, K+ - 9 meq/L. Most likely diagnosis is :**
A. Primary hypothyroidism
B. Congenital adr. hyperplasia
C. Panhypopituitarism
D. Pyloric stenosis

718. **Ir primary adrenal hyperplasia, incorrect is :**
A. Hyponatremia
B. Hypokalemia
C. Hypernatremia
D. Water retention

Ans.	711. A	712. B	713. C	714. B	715. C	716. C
	717. B	718. A				

719. **Which is not a feature of hypothyroid :**
A. Delayed bone age
B. Delayed puberty
C. Altered upper lower segment ratio
D. Short metacarpals in hand

720. **Which of the following statements regarding sex steroid metabolism is not correct ?**
A. All steroid hormones are synthesised from cholesterol
B. Progesterone can be converted into estradiol
C. Estrdiol can be converted into progesterone
D. Testosterone can be converted into estradiol

721. **Which of the following are true of congenital hypothyroidism ?**
1. The child has stunted growth
2. Constipation is common
3. Mental development is subnormal
4. Bone age corresponds to chronological age

Select the correct answer using the codes given below :
A. 1 and 3 B. 2,3 and 4
C. 1,2 and 4

722. **Foetal distress in diabetic mother is caused by all except :**
A. Oral hypoglycemic agents B. Insulin
C. Analgesics D. Sedatives

723. **An infant with an enlarged clitoris may have been born to a mother who received the following except :**
A. Progesterone B. Adrenocortical steroids
C. Testosterone D. Stilbesterol

724. **ACTH secretion is highest during :**
A. Noon B. Evening
C. Morning D. Night

725. **Acromegaly is due to excess of :**
A. ICAM-3 B. GH
C. Somatomedian C D. ILGF

726. **MC enzyme defect in congenital Adr. hyperplasia :**
A. 21-hydroxylase B. 17 hydroxylase
C. 17 Desmolase D. 11-beta hyperoxylase

W727. **A male pseudohermaphrodite child of 46 XY karyotype presents with B.P. 110/80 mmHg. Most likely enzyme deficiency is :**
A. 21 hydroxylase B. 17 alpha hydroxylase
C. 11 hydroxylase D. 3-beta hydroxylase

Ans.	719. D	720. C	721. D	722. B	723. D	724. B
	725. B	726. A	727. B,D			

728. An 11-year-old child, who is mentally and physically retarded with delayed bone age had wormian calcifications in the epiphyses on X-ray. The probabale diagnosis :

A. Hypopituitarism B. Hypothyroidism
C. Malnutrition D. Hypoadrenalism

729. In neonatal screening programme for detection of congenital hypothyroidism, the ideal place and time to collect the blood sample for TSH estimation is :

A. Cord blood at time of birth.
B. Heal pad blood at the time of birth.
C. Heal pad blood on 4 day of birth.
D. Peripheral venous blood on 28 day.

730. Child with recurrent hypoglycemic attacks and hepatomegaly is likely to have :

A. von Gierke disease B. Tetralogy of Fallot
C. Neonatal hepatitis D. Neonatal diabetes

731. Disproportionaste dwarfism occurs in :

A. Hypothyroidism
B. Growth hormone deficiency
C. Achondroplasia
D. Laron dwarf

732. Following is not a true feature of short stature following hypopituitarism :

A. Children are short at birth
B. Proportional dwarfism
C. Bone age is significantly delayed
D. Intelligence is usually normal

733. The following is not true regarding Laron's syndrome :

A. HGH levels are decreased
B. Somatomedin levels are decreased
C. Autosomal recessive inheritance
D. Shows clinical features of pituitary dwarfism

734. Symptoms seen in infants with hypoglycaemia include all except :

A. Cyanosis B. Apnoea
C. Convulsions D. Persistent hunger

735. Major cause of death in diabetics having onset in early childhood is :

A. Cardiac lesions B. Renal microangiopathy
C. Pneumonia D. Hypertensive encephalopathy

Ans.	728. B	729. A	730. A	731. C	732. A	733. A
	734. D	735. B				

736. **Which of the following X-ray finding in a newborn infant would be most suggestive of hypothyroidism ?**
A. Osteoporosis
B. Epiphyseal dysgenesis
C. Prominent thymic shadow
D. Absence of ossification of hamate bone

737. **Which of the following is associated with increased sweat electrolytes ?**
A. Glycogen storage disease
B. Adrenal insufficiency
C. Diabetes insipidus
D. All of the above

738. **Precocious puberty is seen in :**
A. Hyperthyroidism
B. Addison's disease
C. McCune Albright syndrom
D. Neuroblastoma

739. **Which is not associated with tetany?**
A. Seizures
B. Carpopedal spasm
C. Fixed pupils
D. Laryngospasm

740. **Hyperthyroid children excrete increased amounts of all, except :**
A. Tryptamine
B. Tyramine
C. Phenylalanine
D. Catecholamines

741. **A primary manifestation of vaospresin deficiency results from :**
A. Loss of phosphate in urine
B. Loss of potassium in urine
C. Loss of sodium in urine
D. Loss of solute free water

742. **Water tolerance test is useful in differentiating the short stature as a result of :**
A. Hypopituitarism
B. Gonadal dysgenesis
C. Primordial dwarfism
D. Mild hypothyroidis

743. **In evaluating a child with short stature, birth weight is often low in a patient with :**
A. Gonadal dysgenesis
B. Hypopituitarism
C. Hypothyroidism
D. Consittutional delay

744. **The chief presenting complaint of infants with idiopathic hypopituitarism is :**
A. Short stature
B. Headache
C. Convulsion
D. Visual disturbance

Ans.	736. B	737. D	738. C	739. C	740. C	741. D
	742. A	743. A	744. A			

745. Treatment of thyrotoxicosis is :

A. Subtotal thyroidectomy
B. Subtotal ablation with radioactive iodine
C. Blocking thyroid hormone production by drugs
D. Any of the above

746. All are characteristics of Hashimoto's strauma, except:

A. Variable uptake of I131
B. Marked exophthalmos
C. May be preceded by viral infection
D. 95% patients have circulating antithyroid antibodies

747. A newborn with goitre large enough to cause dyspnoea is best treated with :

A. Thyroidectomy
B. Tracheostomy
C. T3
D. Iodides

748. Goitrogenic substances associated with neonatal goitres include all, except :

A. Sulfonamides
B. Iron containing preparation
C. Thioureas
D. Asthma medications containing iodides

749. Metabolic defects shown by hypothyroid infant are all, except :

A. Carotenemia
B. Sensitivity to barbiturates
C. Polycythemia
D. Impaired GFR

750. Suspicious signs of hypothyroidism in a newborn are all, except :

A. Respiratory distress with feeding
B. Subnormal temperatures
C. Persistent diarrhoea
D. Failure to nurse properly

751. In Pendred's syndrome, there is an association between familial goitre and :

A. Harelip
B. Deaf mutism
C. Cataracts
D. Hypospadias

752. Pendred's syndrome associated with cretinism is due to :

A. Peroxidase defect
B. Failure to concentrate iodine
C. Failure to deiodinate iodotyrosines
D. Failure to form iodotyronines

753. Growth hormone does not effect :

A. Carbohydrate metabolism
B. Phosphorus levels
C. Potassium levels
D. Skeletal maturation

Ans.	**745. D**	**746. B**	**747. C**	**748. B**	**749. B**	**750. C**
	751. B	**752. A**	**753. D**			

754. **Adrenocortical insufficiency in infancy usually does not exhibit :**
A. Metabolic acidosis B. Hyperkalemia
C. Hypernatremia D. Poor feeding

755. **Biochemical finding associated with deficiency of 21-hydroxylase in congenital adrenal hyperplasia usually include :**
A. Increase in oestrogens
B. Decrease in ACTH
C. Decrease in testosterone
D. Decreased total 17-ketosteroids

756. **The Commonest cause of congenital hypothyroidism :**
A. Thyroid dysgenesis B. Pendred syndrome
C. Defective release D. Deficiency of deiodinase

757. **Changes associated with adrenocortical tumours include all, except :**
A. Clitoral atrophy
B. Pubic hair development
C. Rugation of labia majora
D. Stippling and pigmentation of scrotum

758. **Hypercorticalism of the adrenal gland is characterised by all of the following except :**
A. Sodium retention B. Hypertension
C. Gluconeogenesis D. Hypotension

759. **Peripheral utilization of glucose is increased in the following :**
A. Pancreatic tumours
B. Tumours of mesothelial origin
C. Prediabetic state
D. All the above

760. **What is the best line of therapy for Cushing's disease :**
A. ACTH B. Cortisone
C. Adrenalectomy D. Hypophysectomy

761. **Virilisation of females is present in all of the following except :**
A. 21 β-hydroxylase deficiency
B. 11 β-hydroxylase deficiency
C. 12 β-hydroxylase deficiency
D. 17 α-hydroxylase deficiency

762. **In cretinism all of the following are seen except :**
A. Mental retardation B. Obesity
C. Sexual infantilism D. Hypoglycemia

763. **Congenital hypothyroidism is diagnosed most early by :**
A. ↑ RAIU B. ↑ TSH
C. T3 levels D. PBI

Ans.	754. C	755. A	756. A	757. A	758. D	759. D
	760. C	761. D	762. C	763. B		

764. For Cushing syndrome in children, best test is :

A. Dexamethasone suppression test
B. ACTH levels
C. CT Scan
D. Steroid assays

765. In the case of male infertility under which one of the following conditions is hormonal therapy indicated ?

A. Hypopituitary hypogonadism
B. Aspermia
C. Retrograde ejaculation
D. Impotency

766. Tetany may be seen with all except :

A. Hypocalcaemia
B. Hypomagnesemia
C. Acidosis
D. Alkalosis

767. Differentiation between Down's syndrome and Cretinism is :

A. Wide set eyes
B. Eyebrows elevated
C. Short neck and fatty appearance
D. Hair growth line recessed

768. In Hyperparathyroidism seen in :

	Ca^+	PO_4^-
A.	↑	↓
B.	↑	↑
C.	↓	↓
D.	↓	•

769. Features of congenital hypothyroidism are following except :

A. Delayed puberty
B. Disproportionate upper lower segment ratio
C. Normal bone age in comparison to height age
D. Short metacarpals

770. Not seen in Reye's syndrome is :

A. Bilirubin more than 3 mg%
B. Aminoaciduria
C. Hypoglycemia
D. Seizures

771. Diabetes insipidus in children may result from all except :

A. A sex-linked dominant genetic disease of the kidneys
B. Hand-Schuller-Christian disease
C. Head injuries
D. Hyperinsulinemia

Ans. **764. D** **765. C** **766. C** **767. A** **768. A** **769. D** **770. A** **771. D**

772. **Hypoglycemia in children may result from following except :**
A. Glucose-6-phosphatase deficiency
B. Hypersensitivity to an amino acid leucine
C. Adrenal insufficiency
D. Islet cell insufficienc

773. **Deficiency of growth hormone leads to :**
A. Delayed fusion of epiphysis
B. Proportionate dwarfism
C. Acromegally
D. Mental retardation

774. **Suppression of lactation is indicated in all except :**
A. Neonatal death
B. Mid trimester abortion
C. IDDM
D. Lithium administration

775. **Milk let down reflex is initiated by ———— hormone :**
A. Oxytocin
B. Oestrogen
C. Prolactin
D. Progesterone

776. **Consider the following features :**
1. Infantile external genitalia
2. Chromosomal defect
3. Primary amenorrhoea
4. Decreased urinary gonadotrophins

Features of Turner's syndrome include :
A. 1,2,3
B. 1,3,4
C. 1,2,4
D. 2,3,4

777. **Dietary treatment of galactosaemia :**
A. Must be continued life long
B. Can be relaxed after puberty
C. Involves delayed weaning
D. Ensures normal intellectual development if started in the first week of life
E. Is best monitored by liver fuction tests

778. **Pelvis showing a characteristic appearance acetabular roof is a feature of :**
A. Down's syndrome
B. Cretinism
C. Gargoylism
D. Morquio disease

779. **True about Klinefelter's syndrome is :**
A. Mental retardation
B. Short stature
C. Chromosomal pattern XO
D. Cubitus valgus

780. **Side effects of corticosteroids include, all, except :**
A. Cataracts
B. Hypoglycaemia
C. Growth retardation
D. Pseudotumour cerebri

Ans.	772. D	773. B	774. C	775. A	776. A	777. A
	778. D	779. A	780. B			

781. Endorine status of the newborn exhibits :

A. High calcium and low phosphorus

B. High PBI and BEI in first weeks

C. High production of ADH

D. All of the above

782. Diabetes mellitus in children most often requires and can be controlled by :

A. Restricted carbohydrate in the diet

B. Oral hypoglycaemic drugs

C. Dietary restriction and oral hypoglycaemic drugs

D. Insulin without dietary restrictions

E. Insulin and some restriction of dietary sugars

783. Infants of diabetic mothers may exhibit the following except :

A. Low blood sugar

B. Low blood calcium

C. Low insulin blood levels

D. Increased proportion of body fat

784. Obesity is associated with :

A. Frolich's syndrome

B. Prader Willi syndrome

C. Laurence-Moon-Biedl syndrome

D. All of the above

785. Upper and lower portion of body disproportion with growth retardation is characteristically seen in :

A. Down's syndrome

B. Turner's syndrome

C. Congenital hypothyroidism

D. Cerebral palsy

786. Familial polyostosis, precocious puberty and pigmenta-tion, the diagnosis is :

A. Cretinism B. Tuberóus sclerosis

C. McCune Albright syndrome D. Toxoplasma infection

787. Nutritional dwarfism is due to :

A. Acute undernutrition

B. Past and persistent malnutrition

C. Chronic malnutrition

D. Kwashiokar

Ans.	**781. B**	**782. E**	**783. C**	**784. D**	**785. C**	**786. C**
	787. C					

788. Which of the following is a feature of Hypothyroid certinism?

A. Deafness with facial palsy
B. Goitre with focal seizures
C. Blindness with mental retardation
D. Goitre with facial palsy

789. Treatment of choice in childhood thyrotoxicosis :

A. Surgery
B. Lugol's iodine
C. Carbimazole
D. Radio iodine

790. Consider the following :

1. Small for date baby
2. Large for date baby
3. Erythroblastosis fetalis
4. Birth asphyxia

Which of these clinical settings predispose(s) to neonatal hypoglycemia ?

A. 1 only
B. 1 and 3
C. 2, 3 and 4
D. 1,2 3 and 4

791. A 13 year old boy has bilateral gynaecomastia. His height is 1.48 cm, weight 58 kg; the sexual maturity rating is tage 2. The gynecomastia is most likely due to :

A. Prolactinoma
B. Testicular tumor
C. Pubertal gyncomastia
D. Chronic liver disease

792. A 9 year old boy presents with growth retardation and propensity to hypoglycemia. Physical examination reveals short stature, micropenia, increased fat and high-pitched voice. The skeletal survey reveals bone age of 5 years. Which of the following is most appropriate diagnosis?

A. Malabsorption
B. Growth hormone deficiency
C. Adrenal tumor
D. Thyroxin dficiency

Ans. 788. A 789. A 790. A 791. C 792. B

EXPLANATIONS OF MCQ's

4. Pre prosomatostatin is processed to two peptides somatostatin 14 and somatostatin 28. Somatostatin is found in various parts of brain where it appararently functions as a neurotransmitter, with effects sensory input, locomotor activity and cognitive function. In hypothalamus, it is growth hormone-inhibiting hormone secreted into portal hypophyseal vesels; in endocrine pancreas, it inhibits insulin secretion and in GIT, it is inhibitory hormone.

   It also results in hypertension

14. There is fall in BMR & depression or psychosis

17. Prolactin releasing hormone has been postulated to exist but not yet fully identified

18. Corticosteroids and not oestrogens produce diabetes mellitus

22. In diabetes insipidus, percentage of filtered water reabsorbed in 87.1% whereas in normal, it is 98.7% absorption. Urine volume is 23.3 L/d in diabetes insipidus whereas in normal it is 2.4 L/d. Urine concentration (mosm/Kg H2O) in diabetes insipidus is 30 whereas in normal, it is 290. There is 20.9 L/d loss of water in excess of solute.

29. There is hyperventilation and fall of ionized calcium.

32. Sertoli cells secrete androgen-binding protein (ABP), inhibin and MIS. They do not synthesize androgens but they contan aromatase (CYp 19), the enzyme responsible for conversion of androgens to estrogens. They can produce estrogens.

37. Aldosterone secretion is increased by

Glucocorticoid secretion also ↑ ed	*Glucocorticoid secretion unaffected*
Surgery	High potassium intake
Anxiety	Low sodium intake
Physical trauma	Constriction of IVC in thorax
Hemorrhage	Standing secondary hyperaldoseronism (in CHF, ARF, Cirrhosis)

39. Cholesterol level rises in thyroxine deficiency (in myxedema)

43. Prolactin inhibitory hormone is Dopamine.

48. In myxoedema, BMR falls

51. Cushing's syndrome is an important cause of hypertension.

53. Hepatic glucose output is increased, producing hyperglycemia. the response to an injection of epinephrine is an initial glycogenolysis follwed by a rise in hepatic glycogen content.

58. Insulin is a polypeptide

65. It is appropriate to check its fasting levels around this time.

74. Cholecystokinin-Pancreozymin is secreted by cells in the mucosa of upper small intestine.

78. Spironolactone (aldosterone antagonist) is used in treatment of oedema in cirrhosis.

86. Cholesterol -> Pregnenolone->17 alpha-> hydroxyprogesterine

↓ ↓ ↓

Progesterone->17 alpha-hydroxy->Progesterone ->Androstenedione

↙

Dihydrotestosterone <———————Testosterone

92. The existence of various natriuretic hormones has been postulated for some time. Two of these are secreted by the heart. the first natriuretic hormone isolated from heart was atrial natriuretic peptide (ANP) with a characteristic 17-amino acid ring. Second is brain natriuretic peptide (BNP) which contains 32 aminoacids and there is C-type natriuretic peptide (CNP) which contains 22 aminoacids.

100. Triglycerides level may rise in thyroxine deficiency

106. In liver 25 dihydroxycholecalciferol in formed whear 1, 25 derivative is formed in kidney.

108. LH stimulates the Leydig cells which involves increased formation of cAMP via the serpentine LH receptor and G8. Cyclic AMP increases the formation of cholesterol from cholesteryl esters and the conversion of cholesterol to pregnenolone via the activation of protein kinase A. The testosterone secretion rate is 4-9 mg/d (13.9-31.33 mmol/d) in normal adult males.

110. Ostriol is main hormone of pregnancy

119. They secrete calcitonin. See Ques. 123

123. Calcitonin is secreted by para follicular cells which are also known as clear or C-cells.

129. ACTH increases secretion of glucocorticoids. The morning plasma ACTH cencentration in a healthy resting human is about 25 pg/mL (5.5 pmol/L).

136. It more active than T4

144. Like other steroids, estrogens combine with protein receptors in the nucleus and the complex binds to DNA, promoting formation of new proteins which modify cell function.

148. Osteoporosis is common after menopause

157. Some of the hormones produced are gastrin, cholecystokinin-pancreozymin, secretin, GIP, VIP, Motilin, Neurotensin, Substance P, GRP, Bombesin, Somatostatin, Guanylin, Urogastrone etc.

159. Somatostatin inhibits secretion of GH, gastrin, VIP, GIP, secretion and motilin.

165. • The hormones of the post-pituitary gland (ADH and oxytocin) are synthesised in the cell bodies of magnocellular

neurons in the supraoptic and para-ventricular nuclei.

- Vasopressin and oxytocin each have a characteristic neurophysin ass. with them in the granules in the neurons that secrete them, neurophysin II in case of vasopressin and neurophysin I in case of oxytocin.
- ADH secretion is enhanced by angiotensin II, prostaglandins, histamine, neuropeptide Y and Ach and is inhibited by GABA and ANP.
- ADH responsive water channel is collecting ducts of kidney is aquaporin-2.

166. Sertoli cells have receptors for FSH which stimulate by FSH and secrete the inhibin.

Sertoli

- Large, complex glycogen - containing cells.
- They provide nutrition to the developing sperm cells.
- They phagocytoze the injured or dead sperm cells.
- They are the basis of blood testis barrier.
- They secrete *androgen-binding protein (ABP), inhibin and MIS.*
- They do not synthesize androgens, but they contain *aromatase*, the enzyme responsible for conversion of androgens to estrogens and they can produce estrogens.

Note:

- *ABP* probably functions to maintain a high, stable supply of androgen in tubular fluid.
- *Inhibin* inhibits FSH secretion.
- *MIS* causes regression of the mullerian ducts in males during fetal life.

167. **Control of the onset of puberty**

- The factors that normally activate or restrain the hypothalamic neurons responsible for GnRH secretion are unknown.
- It is clear that GnRH is the major, if not the only, hormone responsible for the onset and progression of puberty.
- During the period from birth to puberty, a neural mechanism is operating to prevent the normal pulse release of GnRH. The nature of the mechanism inhibiting the GnRH pulse generator is unknown.

- Controversely, opioid peptide such as the enkephalins and β-endorphin reduce the frequency of Gn RH pulses.
- The release of hypothalamic GnRH is also inhibited by melatonin (samson wright).
- Norepinephrine and possibly epinephrine in the hypothalamus increase GnRH pulse frequencies.

169. INHIBIN :

- Factor of testicular origin that inhibits FSH secretion
- Source - Testes in Men

170. "Calcium lowers the circulating calcium and phosphate level. It exerts its calcium lowering effect by inhibiting bone resorption. This action is direct, and calcitonin inhibits the activity of osteoclast.".

- Ovarian Follicles in women

171. "Thyroid hormones enter cells and binds to thyroid receptor in the nuclei. "The hormone receptor complex binds to DNA via zinc finger.

- Nuclear receptors for thyroid hormones are members of the superfamily of hormone sensitive nuclear transcription factor.

I. **Hormones having intracellular receptors**

1. Throid hormones
2. Glycocorticoids
3. Mineralocorticoids
4. Sex hormones

II. **Hormones having cell membrane receptors**

a. Second messenger : cAMP

1. CRH
2. ACTH
3. TSH
4. FSH
5. LH
6. MSH
7. ADH
8. Calcitonin
9. PTH
10. Catecholamines
11. Glucagon
12. hCG

b. Second messenger : cGMP

1. ANF
2. No

c. Second messernger : Calcium/Phosphatidylinositol (or both)

1. TRH
2. GnRH
3. ADH (Vasopressor action)
4. Oxytocin
5. Catecholamines
6. CCK
7. Gastrin

d. Second messanger; Kinase/Phosphatase

1. GH
2. Prolactin
3. Insulin

172. Metformin is having short half life.

174. Long term steroid treatment results in resorption of bone matrix.

175. Sulphonamides increases the activity of oral contraceptives

178. Ultra lente insulin has longest duration of action.

181. Danazol is an orally active ethisterone derivative having mild androgenic, anabolic and progestational activity.

184. Prednisolone is having greatest antiinflammatory activity.

187. Oestrogens are secreted by the ovary. It has actions over sex organs, secondary sex organs and metabolic effects. Oestrogens bind to specific cytoplasmic receptors in target cells and r

190. Guanethidine is taken up into the adrenergic nerve endings by active amine transport.egulate protein synthesis.

192. Desmopressin is the drug of choice in diabetes insipidus. Dose is individualized by measuring 24 hour urine volume.

193. Mifepristone is a 19-norsteroid with potent competitive antiprogestational and significant antiglucocorticoid activity. It is used for termination of pregnancy, contragestational, induction of labour and in Cushing's syndrome.

199. Hypoglycemia is not an adverse effect of cortisone therapy

205. Bromocriptine is used in hyperprolactenemia, Suppression of lactation and breast engorgement, acromegaly and parkinsonism.

206. Oral hypoglycemic agents stimulate insulin secretion and increases the senstivity of cells to insulin.

208. Dichlorophen is not an oral hypoglycemic agent.

211. In pituitary insufficiency, adrenal steroids are contraindicated.

214. Biguanides can cause lactic acidosis.

217. Lithium causes hypothyroidism.

220. Glibenclamide is 2nd generation sulphonylurea.

223. Prednisone is the treatment of choice in Querian thyroiditis.

225. Rifampicin increases the activity of oral contraceptives.

228. Clomiphene citrate is mainly used in treatment of infertility, 50 mg once daily for 5 days starting from 5th day of cycle. Its other uses are in vitro fertilisation and oligospermia.

232. Sulphonylurea does not inhibit release of insulin.

234. Hydrocortisone is the drug of choice for Addison's disease.

237. Corticosteroids maintain fluid balance, cardio- vascular and energy substrate homeostasis and functional status of skeletal muscles and nervous system.

241. Side effects of clomiphene are polycystic ovaries, multiple pregnancy, hot flushes, gastric upset, vertigo & allergic dermatitis.

246. Thiouracil causes agronulocytosis.

249. Catecholamines are immediately released after injury.

250. Glucose absorption is blocked by buformin.

257. Chlorpropamide metabolism is enhanced by ethyl alcohol.

258. Dexamethasone is 30 times potent than cortisone.

261. Affective disorders are most common side effects of prolonged use of steroids.

264. Cortisone and dexamethosone are effective in the absence of a functioning adrenal gland.

271. Dose of levothyronine is 0.1 mg.

275. Insulin from human is preferred because allergic reactions are less.

277. Calcitonin is given in hypercalcemic states like hyperparathyroidism, hypervitaminosis D etc. and postmenopausal osteoporosis.

280. Glucagon receptors are on cell membrane.

286. Immunosuppresive effect of cortisone is attributed to its ability to produce **lymphopenia.**

291. In diabetic coma, drug of choice is crystalline insulin.In diabetic coma, drug of choice is crystalline insulin.

296. Thyroxine does not effect the metabolic rate of brain.

299. Tamoxifen binds to oestrogen receptors.

318. Androgens and all other steroidal hormone, act through receptors.

321. • α-glycosidase inhibitors do not stimulate insulin release and therefore do not result in hypoglycemia

Alpha-glucosidase inhibitors

- It competitively inhibits the a-glucosidase enzyme in the gut which digest dietary starch and sucrose
- Two of these drugs-Acarbose and miglitol are available for clinical use
- It shows down and decreases digestion and absorption of polysaccharides and sucrose
- Regular use tends to lower HbA_1c, body weight and serum triglyceride
- The principal adverse effect is flatulence and diarrhoea
- When acarbose is given alone, there is no risk of hypoglycemia
- It may be used as an adjuvant to diet (with or without sulfonyl urea) in obese diabetics
- They reduce postprandial plasma glucose levels in type 1 DM and type 2 DM subjects
- They typically are used in combination with other oral hypoglycemic agents and/or insulin

322. **Biguanides**

- They do not cause insulin release, but presence of some insulin is essential for their action.
- Cause little or no hypoglycemia in non-diabetic subjects
- Suppress hepatic gluconeogenesis and glucose output from liver (major action)
- Enhance binding of insulin to its receptors
- Promote peripheral glucose utilization by enhancing anaerobic glycolysis
- Inhibit intestinal absorption of glucose
- Lactic acidosis is more common with phenformin
- It is C/I in hypotensive states, cardiovascular, respiratory, hepatic and renal disease

Sulfonyl ureas

- Increase release of insulin from pancreas (by reducing conductance of ATP sensitive K^+ channels)
- A minor action is reducing glucagon and increasing somatostatin release
- They sensitize the target tissue (esp. liver) to action of insulin due to increase in number of insulin receptors

Note

Oral hypoglycaemics are indicated only in uncomplicated NIDDM, when not controlled by diet and exercise.

323. * Raloxifene does not reduce hot flushes, vaginal dryness, skin wrinkling, or breast atrophy, it does not improve. Cognition (infact, it increases the hot flush)

* Raloxifene is an selective estrogen receptor modulators (SERMs)

* Tibolone is an SERM whose metabolites have mixed estrogenic, progestogenic, and weak androgenic activity. It is comparable to hormone replacement therapy for the treat ment of climacteric-related complaints (includes hot flushes).

* **Isoflavones** are phytoestrogens that bind weakly to estrogen receptor but have over 80% of estrogen's affinity for estrogen receptor.

* Soy and red clover isoflavones are selective estrogen receptor modulators, which acta as estrogen on bone, brain, and vasculature but have no stimulatory effects upon the uterus or breast.
* Daily intake of 60 gm of isolated soy protein reduces hot flushing by about 455 within 12 weeks. They also improves plasma lipid profile and inhibit development of coronary atherosclerosis in male monkeys.
* **Androgens-** Androgen deficiency contributes to hot flushes loss of lipids and sexual hair, muscle atrophy, and osteoporosis selected women may be treated with low-dose methyltestosterone, which is available in combination with conjugated estrogenis.

328. Embryonically the thyroid anlage begins in the region of foramen caecum at the base of tongue and as the gland develops, it descends to its definitive location in the anterior neck. Ramnants of this tract may persist producing cysts, 1-4 cm in diameter, that may be lined with stratified squamous epithelium when cyst is near base of tongue or pseudostratified columnar epithelium who cyst is in lower locations.

343. In adrenals, diffuse hyperplasia is found in 60 to 70% cases of Cushing's syndrome. Both glands are enlarged. Nodular hyperplasia accounts for 15-20% cases of Cushing's syndrome.

350. In Hashimoto's thyroiditis in goitrous form, there is extensive replacemnt of underlying parenchyma by lymphocytes, plasma cells, immunoblasts, macrophages, sometimes with formation of lymphoid germinal center. Hurthle cells or oncocytes may also be seen.

356. In MEN-I (Wermer's syndrome), Pituitary, Parathyroid, Pancreatic islets, Adrenal and thyroid are involved. There is 11q 11-13 mutant gene locus whereas in MEN-II (Sipple's syndrome) Parathyroid, Adrenal and thyroid are involved. Mutant gene locus is on chromosome 10 (near centromere). In MEN IIb or III, parathyroid, adrenal thyroid. extraendocrine changes (mucocutaneous ganglioneuromas and marfanoid habitus).

365. In haemochromatosis, pancreas becomes pigmented, heart is often enlarged and has hemosiderin granules within myocardial fibres, skin is pigmented, haemosiderin deposition in joint synovial linings and testes may be small and atrophic but are not usually significantly pigmented in most common cause of secondary haemochromatosis are the severe anemias associated with ineffective erythropoisis, fully developed cases exhibit, micronodular cirrhosis (most cases), DM (75-80%) and skin pigmentation (75-80%).

369. Appendix is the most common site of gut carcinoid tumors followed by small intestine (ileum), rectum, stomach and colon.

378. There is male pseudohermaphroditism, The most common form called complete androgen insensitivity syndrome (testicular feminization) results from mutations of gene for androgen receptors. This gene is located at Xq 11-Xq 12; hence this disorder is X-linked recessive.

387. Paraneoplastic, aging, androgen therapy and other drugs may produce.

394. There is low serum calcium but PTH is raised whereas in primary and tertiary types, Ca and PTH are raised. Mal absorption, osteomalacia and rickets are other important causes.

400. Myxoedema is associated with decreased level of consciousness, decreased Body temp.

410. Increased Calcitonin is the main abnormality in addition to ACTH and Prostaglandin, It arises from parafollicular 'c' cells.

411. It is seen in 30-40 years. It most often spreads to bone, lungs and brain.

417. Sexual dysfunction can be produced by follwoing drugs :

Impaired ejaculation	*Decreased libido & impotence*	*Impairment of spermatogenesis or oogenesis*	*Priapism*
Bethanidine	Beta blockers	Cytotoxic drugs drugs	Trazodone
Debrisoquin	Clonidine		
Guanethidine	Diuretics		
Thioridazine	HIV protease inhibitors		
Lithium			
Major tranquilizers			
Methyldopa			
OCP			
Sedatives.			

420. In contrast to Pigmentation of Addisons disease a striking degree of pallor is usually present because of lack of melanin in the skin.

429. It is due to premature activation of HPA axis.

444. These are features of Hypothyroidism except: Pretibial myxoedema is a feature of Graves disease.

450. Glycosylated Hb-I is a result of non enzymatic addition of sugar moiety to valine of Beta chain.

455. There may be wide pulse pressure, sinus tachycardia, atrial fibrillation, systolic murmurs, increased intensity of apical first sound, cardiac enlargement and failure. A to-and-fro high pitched sound is heard in pulmonic area and may simulate pericardial rub called Means—Lerman Scratch.

460. Other conditions associated with SIADH are —Ca lung (small cell), Pancreas, duodenum, ureter, Bladder, prostate, lymphoma, Mesothelioma, Polio, T.B., Pneumonia.

— Drugs-Narcotics, Phenothazines, Carbamazepine, TCA, MAO inhibitors, Vincristine, Cyclophosphamide, NSAIDS.

— Meningitis, encephalitis, Head injury.

464. High serum TSH level is earliest indicator to compensate for decreased in T3, T4. T3 does not discriminate between euthyroid and hypothyroid and should not be measured.

471. Polyuria, excessive thirst and polydipsia are invariably present. Desmopressin, Pitressin, Chlorpropamide, Clofibrate, Carbamazepine have been used for treatment.

473. Galactorrhoea can be produced by domperidone, methyldopa, metoclopramide, phenothiazines, reserpine, risperidone, tricyclic antidepresants.

476. In osteoporosis, serum Alkaline phosphatase also remains normal.

481. With treatment TSH tends to fall.

489. This remains high in thyrotoxicosis

500. But in nephrotic syndrome quantity of Protein is decreased in serum & hence sufficient protein is not available for binding.

508. The causes of Tetany includes.

Malabsorption, osteomalacia, Hypopara thyroidism, CRF, Excessive vomiting, excessive oral alkali, Hyperventilation, Pri. hyperaldosteronism.

515. It is seen in Type I DM. About half of the patients develop this complication. It may remain silent for long periods (10-15 years). Progression of renal diseases is accelerated by hypertension

525. It is the commonest cause of hypercalcemia.

534. Hypoglycemia can be produced by ACE inhibitors, insulin, octreotide, oral hypoglycemics, pentamidine and quinine.

545. Subacute thyroiditis is also called de Quervains thyroiditis. Symptoms are pain in Thyroid, jaw, parotid or ear, Iodine uptake is low because damaged follicles are unable to trap Iodine.

565. Thyroid dysfunction can be produced by drugs eg acetazolamide, amiodarone, Bromsulfophthalein, chlorpropamide, clofibrate, colestipol and nicotinic acid, dimercaprol, gold salts, lithium, oral contraceptives, phenindione, phenothiazines, phenylbutazone, phenytoin, sulfonamides, tolbutamide

567. There is pigmentation on exposed and friction prone areas.

583. A loading dose of 10-20 units of unmodified Insulin is given I/M immediately followed by 4-6 units hourly thereafter I/M or I/V infusions. The blood glucose should fall by 3-6 mmol per hour.

590. It indicates pituitary dysfunction.

599. Gynaecomastia can be produced by calcium channel antagonists, clomiphene, digitalis (painful gynaeconastia), estrogens, ethionamide, griseofulvin, INH, methyldopa, phenytoin, reserpine, spironalactone, testosterone.

605. Addisonian like syndrome can be produced by busulfan, etomidate and kitocanazole

634. It is the commonest cause.

639. Cerebral mucomycosis is also common in diabetics.

662. In diabetic ketoacidosis, insulin is treatment of choice.

663. Diabetes mellitus is not related to central causes.

665. In diabetic ketoacidosis, insulin is treatment of choice.

666. It indicates pituitary dysfunction.

682. Read pre-receptor, receptor and post-receptor resistance of insulin (Insulin resistance is defined as more than 200 units required per day).

683. Also called granulomatous or giant cell thyroiditis, is viral in origin. Two laborator findings —high ESR and a depressed RAIU are characteristic. In mild cases aspirin and in severe cases steroids alongwith propranolol are used.

684. Rather hypoglycemia may be seen in adrenocortical insufficiency (Addison's disease) Hyponatremia hyperkalemia and hypercalcemia may be seen.

685. Urinary VMA and metanephrines are useful in diagnosis.

686. Profuse sweating, weight loss, sinus tachycardia sinus bradycardia, SVT or ventricular premature contractions, angina and Mi may be seen. Fatal paroxysms may be induced by opiates, histamine ACTH, saralsin and glucagon.

687. There is lack of streking fluid retention in most instances of primary aldosteronism (Conn's syndrome).

688. Hypertension is also seen.

689. Severe hypothyroidism occassionally causes impaired release of GH and ACTH after appropriate stimuli.

700. * **Noonan syndrome** - Male to male transmission based on autosomal dominent gene with variable expressivity. This gene, clinical has been mapped to chromosome 12q.

* Clinical manifestations - The most common abnormalities are short stature, webbing of the neck, pectus carinatum or pectus excavatum, cubitus valgus, right sided congenital heart disease and characteristic focies.

* Cardiac defect is most often pulmonary valvular stenosis; others are hypertrophic cardiomyopathy and atrial septal defect,

* Males frequently have cryptorchidism and small testes; there may be hypogonadism or they may be normal.

* In girls sexual maturation usually occurs but is delayed, 2 year on average and premature ovarian failure has also been reported.

701. • Ketone bodies absent in non insulin dependent diabetes mellitus and present in IDDM.

• Oral hypoglycemics are indicated only in uncomplicated NIDDM, when not controlled by diet and exercise (KDT).

703. Gynaecomastia

Glandular enlargement of the male breast that may be tender and is often asymmetric or unilateral.

- Laboratory investigation of unclear cases should include the following:

1. Chest X-ray (for metastatic or bronchogenic Ca)
2. Plasma level of prolactin and bHCG
3. Plasma testosterone and LH
4. Serum estradiol is determined but is usually normal
5. Serum TSH and tree thyroxine level
6. Needle biopsy with cytologic examination

704. **Jod–Basedow effect**

Iodine induce hyperthyroidism may occur in both endemic or sporadic multimodular goiters after intake of large amounts of iodine in the diet or in the form of radiographic contrast materials or drugs, esp. amiodarone.

Thyrotoxicosis factitia

It is form of thyrotoxicosis without hyperthyroidism that results from purposeful or inadvertent ingestion of large amounts of thyroid hormone.

Wolff-Chaikoff effect

Iodide–induced goiter with or without hypothyroidism appears to arise from an intrinsic defect in the organic binding mechanism, which permits a persistent Wolff-Chaikoff effect.

Euthyroid patients with grave's disease, esp. after surgery or radioiodine treatment, patient with Hashimoto's disease and normal fetuses are particularly susceptible to iodine-induced goiter.

708. **ACE Inhibitors.** Drugs in this group inhibit the enzyme converting angiotensin I into angiotensin II-*ACE2.* These agents are an increasingly popular choie for initial therapy. They are useful because they not only inhibit the generation of a potent vasoconstrictor (angiotensin II) but also retard the degradation of a potent vasodilator (badykinin), alter prostaglandin production, and can modify the activity of the adrenergic nervous system. They are especially useful in renal or renovascular hypertension and in diabetic patients as well as in accelerated and malignant hypertension.

709. **Multiple Sclerosis is a cause for primary polydipsia (not DI).** Even the table given on CMDT 2004, page 1070 does nto mention multiple sclerosis as the cause of diabetes insipidus.

Causes of Diabetes insipidus -

* Primary Diabetes Insipidus

  Acquired
  - Head trauma
  - Neoplasms
  - Granulomas (Histiocytosis)
  - Infectious (Viral encephalitis)
  - Inflammatory
  - Chemical toxins
  - Vascular
  - Pregnancy
  - Idiopathic

  Congenital malformations Genetic

  Genetic

* Nephrogenic Diabetes inspidus

  Acquired
  - Drugs
  - Lithium
  - Demeclocycline
  - Methoxyflurane
  - Amphotericin B
  - Cisplatin
  - Rifampin
  - Foscarnet
  - Metabolic
  - Obstruction
  - Granulomas
  - Neoplasms
  - Infiltration
  - Pregnancy
  - Idiopathic
  - Genetic

* **Primary Polydipsia -**

  Acquired

* Psychogenic

  Dipsogenic (abnormal thirst)
  - Granulomas
  - Infectious
  - Head trauma
  - Demyelinatio (*Multiple Sclerosis)*
  - Drugs- (Lithium and Carbamazepine)
  - Idiopathic

  Iatrogenic

710. * Androgen Insensitivity Syndrome - Mutations in the androgen receptor (AR) cause resistance to androgen (testosterone, DHT) action or the androgen insensitivity syndrome (AIS).

* AIS is a spectrum of disorders that affects at least 1 in 100, 000 chromosomal males. Because the androgen receptor is x-linked, only males are affected and maternal carriers are phenotypically normal.

* *XY individuals with complete AIS (testicular feminization syndrome) have a female phenotype, normal breast development, a short vagina but no uterus (because MIS production is normal), scanty pubic and axillary hair, and female psychosexual orientation.*

* **Gonadotropins and testosterone levels can be loco, normal or elevated, depending on the degree of androgen resistance and the contribution by estradiol to feedback inhibition of the hypothalmic-pituitary gonadal axis.**

* Most patients present with inguinal herniae (containing testes) in childhood or with primary amenorrhoea in adulthood.

* Gonadectomy is usually performed, as there is a low risk of malignancy, and estrogen replacement is prescribed.

* Partial AIS (Reifenstein syndrome) results from less severe AR mutation.

* Patients often present in infancy with perineoscrotal hypospadias, small cryptorchid testes, and with gynecomastia at the time of puberty.

Other disorder affecting males (46, xy)

* Persistent Mullerian Duct syndrome
* Isolated hypospadias
* Cryptorchidism

711.* Disease Associations in the Multiple Endocrine Neoplasia (MEN) syndromes.

Men 1	Men 2 A	Men 2B
* Parathyroid hyperplasia Adenomas Pheochromocytoma	* Medullary CA of thyroid * Pheochromocytoma	* Medullary CA of thyrodi *
* Islet cell hyperplasia, adenoma or carcinoma	* Parathyroid hyperplasia or adenoma	* Mucosal and gastrointestinal symptoms
* Pituitary hyper-plasia/adenoma	* Cutaneous lichen amylordosis	* Marfanoid features
* Other less common - Foregut carcinoid, disease - Pheochromo-cytoma - subcutaneous or visceral lipoma - dermal angiofibroma or collagenomas	* Hirschsprung	

712* Humoral hypercalcemia of malignancy (HHM) occurs in upto 5 of patients with cancer.

* HHM is most common in cancers of lung, breast, head and neck, genitourinary tract, esophagus and skin and in multiple myeloma and lymphomas.
* There are several humoral causes of HHM but it is most often associated with overproduction of PTHrP.
* **In addition to acting as a circulating humoral factor, many bone diseases (e.g. breast, multiple myeloma) produce PTHrP, leading to local osteolysis and hyper calcemia.**

Paraneoplastic Syndromes caused by Ectopic Hormone production

	Paraneoplastic Syndrome	*Ectopic Hormone*	*Typical Tumor Types*
*	parathyroid hormone Hypercalcemia of malignancy	squameous cell releated protein (PTHrP) 1, 25 dihydroxy vitamin) parathyroid hormone (PHT) (rare), prosta-glandin E2 (PGE2) (rare)	(head, & neck, lung, skin) breast, genitrourinary, gastrointestinal lymphomas, lung, ovary, renal, lung.
*	Syndrome of inappropriate antidiuretic hormone secretion (SIADH)	vasopressin	Lung (squamous, small cell) gastro intestinal, genitourinary ovary
	Cushing's syndrome	Adrenocorticotropic hormone (ACTH)	Lung (small cell, bronchial carcinoid, adenocarcinoma, squamous), thy-mus, pancreatic islet, medullary thyroid carcinoma.

713. "Even patients treated with topical or inhaled steroids may develop clinically significant suppresion of the hypothalamic pituitary - adrenal axis."

- Symptoms usually begin in the first 48 horus after descontrinuation of the steroid medication.

* Secondary adrenal insufficiency can become manifest shortly after the cessation of corticosteroid therapy or months later in a stressful setting such as after an injury or surgical procedure.

* The duration of impairment can be as long as one year after the correction of hypercortisolism.

Secondary hypoadrenalism (adrenocorticotropic hormone deficiency.

- This is a common clinical problem and is most often due to sudden cessation of exogenous glucocorticoul therapy. Such therapy suppresses the hypothalamic-pituitary -adrenal axis with consequent adrenal atrophy, and thes may last for months after stoping glucocorticoid treatment.

- *Adrenal atophy and subsequent deficiency should be expected in any subject who has taken more than the equivallent of 30 mg. of hydrocortisone per day orally (or 7.5 mg/day prednisolone or 0.75 mg/day dexamethasone) for more than 3 weeks.*

714. The new WHO classification will represent the culmination of the ***efforts of the informal international lymphoma study group to adjust the "REAL classification, following an international investigation to test its reproducibility, validity and clinical relevance.***

REAL (Revised European-American Lymphoma) classification is based on the premise that B-cell malignancies are distinct from T-cell malignancies.

International lymphoma study group REAL classification

B-cell neoplasms

I. precursor B-cell neoplasm
II. Peripheral B-cell neoplasm
T-cell and putative NK-cell Neoplasms
I. Precursor T-cell neoplams
II. Peripheral T-cell and NK-cell neoplasms

726. It most often results due to 21 hydroxylase deficiency.

727. Pseudohermaphroditism is also seen in 3 beta hydroxylase deficiency but hypertension is not seen.

738. Puberty before age of 8 years in girls or 9 years in boys is considered precocious puberty. It is central (true) or peripheral (pseudo type).

744. In hypopituitarism, birth weight and height are normal and there is slow growth from a few months after birth (progressive retardation), puberty is delayed and GH levels are low.

751. Pendred syndrome is autosomal recessive and there is congenital deafness and goitre. Hearing loss is usually present at birth and goitre appears at puberty.

756. Goitrous hypothyroidism can result due to dyshormonogenesis, iodine deficiency antithyroid drugs and Hashimoto's disease.

768. Alkaline phosphatase is also raised.

774. It is due to increase in dopamine levels, stimulating prolactin Inhibiting factor.

779. Chromosomal pattern is XXY. Cubitus valgus, XO patterna and short stature are seen in Turner's syndrme.

785. Ratio between upper and lower segment is increased. Child appears short and stocky.

786. It is a diaphyseal disorder like Englemann and Caffey's diseases.

791. During early to mid puberty, approximately two thirds of boys develop various degrees of subareolar hyperplasia of the breasts. *Physiologic pubertal gynecomastia* may involve only one brest, and it is not unusual for both breasts to enlarge at disproportionate rates or at different times. Tenderness of the breast is common but transitory. Spontaneous regression may occur within a few months; it rarely persists longer than 2 yr.